Energy
Boosters
H A N D B O O K

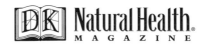

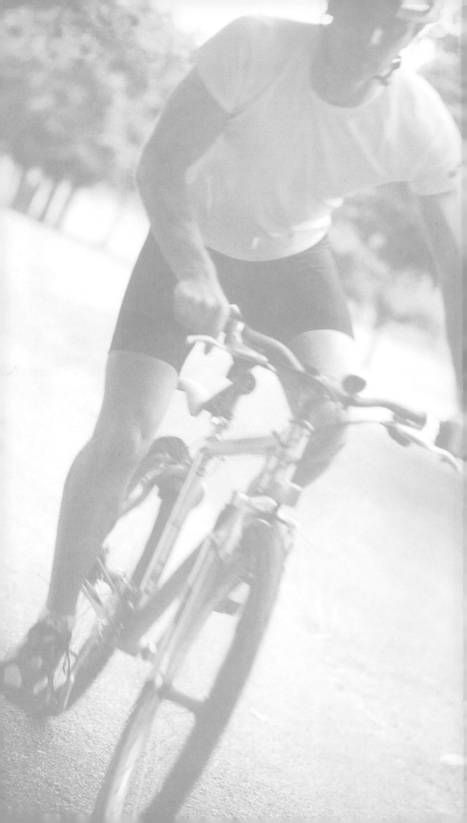

Energy
Boosters
H A N D B O O K

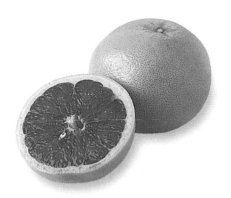

Dr. Sarah Brewer
MA MB BChir

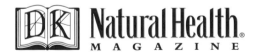

LONDON, NEW YORK, MUNICH,
MELBOURNE, DELHI

Natural Health magazine is the leading publicaton in the field of natural
self-care. For subscription information call 800-526-8440 or visit
www.naturalhealthmag.com. Natural Health® is a registered trademark
of Weider Publications, Inc.

This book was edited by **Jude Garlick** and designed by **Axis Design Editions**

Dorling Kindersley
Senior Editor **Penny Warren**
US Editors **Jill Hamilton, Connie Novis**
Senior Art Editor **Margherita Gianni**
Managing Editor **Stephanie Farrow**
Managing Art Editor **Mabel Chan**
Category Publisher **Daphne Razazan**
DTP Designer **Karen Constanti**
Production Controller **Joanna Bull**

First American Edition, 2002
2 4 6 8 10 9 7 5 3 1
Published in the United States by DK Publishing, Inc.
375 Hudson Street, New York, New York 10014

Copyright © 2002 Dorling Kindersley Limited, London

Text copyright © 2002 Dr. Sarah Brewer

Library of Congress Cataloguing-in-Publication Data
Brewer, Sarah.
Energy boosters handbook: revitalizing techniques to increase energy levels and restore zest for life / Sarah
Brewer.
p.cm. -- (Healing handbooks)
Includes index.
ISBN 0-7894-8442-0 (alk.paper)
1. Dietary supplements-Handbooks, manuals, etc. 2. Nutrition--Handbooks, manuals, etc.
3. Vital force--Handbooks, manuals, etc. 4. Health--Handbooks, manuals, etc. 5. Longevity--
Nutritional aspects--Handbooks, manuals, etc. I. Title. II. Series.
RA776.95.B74 2002
613.2--dc21
2001047930

Color reproduction by GRB, Italy
Printed and bound by South China Printing CO. Ltd., China

While the author has made every effort to provide accurate, up-to-date information at the
time of writing, nutritional and medical science is constantly evolving. You are strongly advised
to consult a medical practitioner if you have symptoms of illness or if you are on conventional
medication and you wish to take dietary supplements or have complementary treatments.

see our complete product line at
www.dk.com

Contents

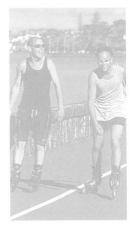
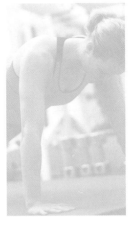
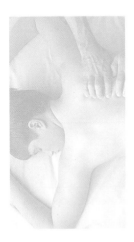

AUTHOR'S
INTRODUCTION

The entire universe is made up of energy. Without a constant supply of it, life could not exist on Earth. Plants absorb energy from sunlight but the energy human beings need is ultimately derived from the food they eat.

THE NATURE OF ENERGY

Energy exists in a number of forms – some of which are visible and obvious and others of which are much more subtle. It has numerous physical properties, many of which are not yet fully understood by scientists. Eastern and Western philosophies view manifestations of energy in a variety of different ways, but most agree that optimum energy levels are equated with optimum health and well-being.

Like plants, humans are able to absorb energy from sunlight, but the only benefit is the conversion of a cholesterol-like molecule in the skin into vitamin D. Otherwise, all the energy needed to fuel metabolism, physical exercise, and brain function is generated from food intake.

A lack of energy is very common. Surveys indicate that at any one time two out of three women, for example, feel excessively tired. Often the main cause is stress. For women, pregnancy and breast-feeding, looking after young children, and the hormone imbalances associated with menstruation or menopause play a major role. Excessive stress drains the adrenal glands and is linked to fatigue and reduced immunity. It also increases the risk of common diseases such as diabetes, coronary artery disease, high blood pressure, stroke, and even cancer. A lack of energy is in itself stressful, so it is important to take steps to try to prevent this vicious cycle from being established.

ESSENTIALS FOR ENERGY

Luckily, several relatively simple dietary and lifestyle changes can help you boost your energy levels. If you eat too many of the wrong foods, you will not obtain sufficient amouns of the vitamins, minerals, and essential fatty acids your body needs.If you eat the right kinds of food, in the right amounts, you will quickly feel more energized. Anyone who has eaten a banana before exercise knows that some foods can pep you up, while others – such as rich, fatty foods – drag you down. If you feel lacking in energy, one of the first things you must examine is your diet. While dietary sources of essential nutrients should be your top priority, many vitamin, mineral, coenzyme, and herbal supplements may provide a much-needed boost when your energy reserves are low. Some supplements provide a purely physical energy boost, while others claim to improve clarity of thought and revitalize the mind. For details of all the nutrients you need and where to find them see pages 26–70.

LOOKING AT LIFE

Next, you must take a look at your lifestyle. Modern work pressures include high levels of stress and long working hours and these soon leave you feeling drained. They weaken

Lifestyle factors, such as getting regular exercise, are significant. Exercise expends energy but it improves energy production.

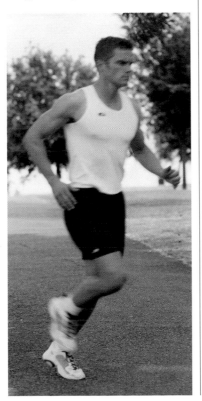

your immunity so that you become susceptible to infections. Taking time out regularly for exercise, rest, relaxation, and rejuvenation is very important. Addressing the sources of stress by improving your time-management, controlling chaos, and boosting your self-esteem and motivation will help stop pressures from building up. Assess your lifestyle on pages 72–109.

A number of complementary techniques claim to affect energy in its different forms to improve your well-being. Aromatherapy, massage, meditation, and visualization, for example, can relax yet at the same time revitalize you. Other options you might like to consider include color therapy, crystal healing, cymatics, reiki or spiritual healing, or perhaps oriental martial-arts-based movement therapies such as t'ai chi ch'uan, qigong, and buqi.

TAKING STEPS

If you think your energy levels are not all they should be, following a program intended to increase physical, mental, and spiritual energy for a few days may provide a good start to revitalizing your diet and lifestyle. You may have an energy deficit linked to a specific problem such as seasonal affective disorder (SAD), disrupted or poor-quality sleep, reduced sexual energy, menopause, or work burnout. In these cases, more specific energy-boosting programs are required. Details of general and particular reenergizing programs can be found on pages 112–23.

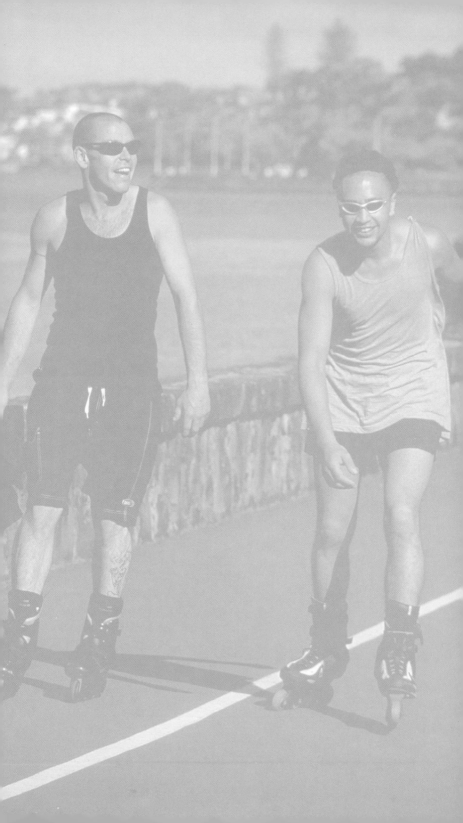

What is Energy?

Diet, fitness, stress levels, mood –
even weather – all have an impact on
how much energy we have. But what
is energy and how is it produced in
the body? This section of the book
explains different concepts of energy,
as understood by western medical
science and some of the world's
traditional healing systems.

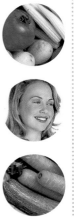

EXPLAINING ENERGY

Energy is the capacity we have to be active in mind, body, and spirit. All the cells in the body need energy to "fuel" their growth, development, and metabolic functions, whether they are used in physical, mental, or sexual activity.

ENERGY IN FOOD

First of all you need to understand how amounts of energy in the body are measured. The standard unit, the calorie, is defined scientifically as the amount of heat energy needed to raise the temperature of 1 g of water by 1° C from 15° C to 16° C. This is also called the standard calorie (cal) and is spelled with a small "c."

People often confuse calories with kilocalories (kcal). The latter are also known as Calories but with a capital "C." One kilocalorie is equivalent to 1,000 calories. Calories are such small units that kilocalories are often used instead. One kilogram (kg) of body fat is equivalent to 7,000 kcal of stored energy.

Different foods provide the body with different amounts of energy. This depends on the chemical structure of their molecules. The body harnesses the energy stored

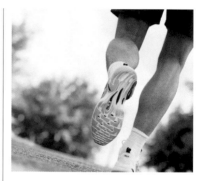

The amount of energy your body needs to generate from day to day depends on your age, how active you are, your fitness level, and the metabolism you have inherited.

in chemical bonds that hold the different molecules together. Carbohydrate and protein provide 4 kcal of energy per gram, but fat is by far the most energy-rich food, supplying 9 kcal of energy per gram.

The energy you need from day to day depends on your physical makeup, including your genetic heritage, as well as lifestyle factors.

YOUR DAILY ENERGY NEEDS

Age	Men	kcal/day	Age	Women	kcal/day
11–14		2,220	11–14		1,845
15–18		2,755	15–18		2,110
19–50		2,550	19–50		1,940
51–59		2,550	51–59		1,900
60–64		2,380	60–64		1,900
65–74		2,330	65–74		1,900
75+		2,100	75+		1,810

HOW IS ENERGY PRODUCED IN THE BODY?

Unlike plants, which use sunlight to generate energy-storage molecules during photosynthesis, human beings and other animals obtain fuel by eating food. Dietary components are then digested, absorbed, and processed in a slow, complex process that generates sources of energy such as fatty acids and glucose.

Energy is produced in the body in mitochondria, tiny structures found in each cell. These resemble rechargeable batteries and are thought to have evolved from primitive bacteria that set up a symbiotic relationship with unicellular organisms millennia ago. Mitochondria contain their own genetic material that programs them to make the enzymes needed during energy-releasing reactions.

In these reactions mitochondria use oxygen, fatty acids, and glucose to generate an energy-rich storage chemical known as ATP (adenosine triphosphate). This readily releases its energy in controlled amounts when it is broken down into ADP (adenosine diphosphate). ADP is usually converted

Muscle cells require a lot of energy, especially when you are working out.

straight back into ATP again, ready for the next round of energy-producing reactions. Fatty acids and glucose are also essential for the regeneration of ATP.

USING ENERGY

Most cells "burn" either fatty acids or glucose to generate ATP but brain cells only use glucose and as soon as blood sugar (glucose) levels start to fall, your mental function rapidly decreases. Resting muscle cells prefer to use fatty acids as fuel, but when you start exercising they switch to using glucose or their own stores of a starchy substance known as glycogen. Muscle cells contain the highest concentration of mitochondria, and regular exercise can both increase their number and size, which is how regular exercise boosts your overall energy levels.

If brain or muscle cells do not receive enough oxygen, glucose, fatty acids, or the vitamins and minerals that are also required for energy-generating processes, you will quickly feel fatigued and lacking in energy. Adequate sleep is also important for energy production, since this is when brain and muscle cells are allowed to rest, repair, rejuvenate, and regenerate so that they can function at their optimum levels.

MAINTAINING ENERGY

The body is such a complex chemical reactor it is surprising that low energy levels are not more common. Humans are so well adapted to life on Earth, however, that most of the time we manage to maintain our energy reserves by paying attention to diet and lifestyle. Healthy eating and the sensible use of food supplements, regular exercise, relaxation periods, and a positive attitude to life all combine to help keep physical, mental, emotional, and sexual energy levels within the optimum range.

Healthy eating means obtaining enough energy, vitamins, minerals, protein, essential fatty acids, and certain other nutrients such as coenzyme Q10 from the diet to meet metabolic needs.

Unless you are confident that you have a nutritious diet, an A–Z-style vitamin and mineral supplement is a good nutritional safety net. Other supplements widely taken to help maintain energy levels include adaptogens, which support the function of the adrenal glands in times of stress. These increase energy production in body cells by optimizing the uptake of oxygen and the removal of cell waste. This encourages cell growth and has been shown in the laboratory to increase cell survival. Adaptogens strengthen, normalize, and regulate body systems. They may also help regulate blood sugar levels and counter the effects of stress.

Paradoxically, although exercise "burns" energy, regular exercise will help boost energy levels by improving cardiovascular fitness and by increasing the number and size of the energy-producing structures (mitochondria) within cells, especially those in muscle cells.

Maintaining a positive outlook on life and taking time out for relaxation and leisure pursuits will also help maintain energy levels.

Every aspect of your lifestyle can affect your energy levels. Combining leisure and exercise is a great way of boosting energy.

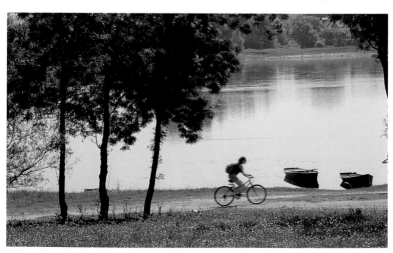

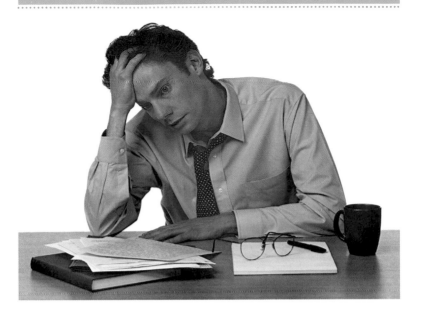

WHY ENERGY LEVELS FALL

The main causes of nonspecific lack of energy – whether mental, physical, or sexual – are stress, overwork, lack of sleep, little or no exercise, and a poor diet that leads to nutritional deficiencies.

Stress drains the adrenal glands and lowers immunity. It rapidly depletes B-group vitamins and increases the need for antioxidants such as vitamins C and E, beta-carotene, and selenium. Stress-busting techniques, from relaxation therapies (such as massage) to spiritually uplifting exercise programs (such as yoga), can help replenish energy. Making sure you have enough restful sleep is vitally important, too.

If you eat too many of the wrong kinds of foods, you will quickly feel bloated, generally slowed down, and fatigued. Research shows, for example, that eating fatty foods for breakfast can make you sluggish

Stress results in nutrient deficiencies which impair the metabolism so less energy is produced and it is used less efficiently.

throughout the morning. If you start the day with a bowl of cereal, in contrast, you will improve your memory function, concentration, recall of new information, and mental performance.

If you skip meals because of lack of time, cut back drastically on eating (for example, if you are trying to lose weight), or eat too many of the wrong kinds of food and not enough of the right ones, energy levels will also soon fall. Important energy-boosting nutrients often in short supply are B-group vitamins, iron, calcium, magnesium, and iodine.

Even the time of the year can affect your energy levels. Seasonal Affective Disorder (SAD) is a form of depression that occurs in the winter months when exposure to natural sunlight is reduced.

CONCEPTS OF ENERGY

Energy can be thought of in a number of ways. In human terms, it is characterized mainly as physical, mental, and spiritual. But more philosphical ideas refer to "life energy," which is responsible for all aspects of our well-being.

ENERGY LINKS

All the different types of energy are interconnected. When levels of one kind are low, levels of the others are usually depleted, too. It is unlikely that you will feel mentally alert or sexually aroused, for example, if you are physically exhausted at the end of a grueling week.

In ancient China, the flow of sexual energy around the body was believed to be fundamental to physical, emotional, and spiritual well-being, and channeling sexual energy was considered the key to immortality. Herbal aphrodisiacs and erotic art were used extensively, not merely to increase pleasure in sex, but as a means of improving all energy levels, vitality, and longevity.

The same concept was embraced by Traditional Chinese Medicine, which considered sexual energy to be the manifestation of an individual's constitutional essence, or *jing*. *Jing* is stored in the kidneys and is responsible for development and reproduction. If *jing* becomes depleted, it leads to recurrent ill-health and premature aging.

In the West, the idea of trying to maintain a balance between physical, emotional, and sexual energy is often neglected, especially by people who live under constant pressure. The more stressed you become, the lower your sex drive will be. Chinese medicine sees this as nature's way of conserving *jing* and considers low libido to be a sign of imbalance and ill-health. Many practitioners recommend that sex is followed by a period of relaxation to allow sexual energy and libido to be replenished.

QI AND MERIDIANS

The ancient, Asian philosophy on which acupuncture is based proposes that a life force flows through the body along channels known as meridians. In China, this vital energy is known as *qi*, while in Japan it is known as *ki*.

There are 12 main meridians, six of which have a *yang* polarity (*see below*) and are associated with hollow organs such as the stomach, and six are *yin* (*see below*), relating mainly to solid organs, for example, the liver. Eight further meridians control these 12. A number of points (acupoints) are located along each meridian. These points are where *qi* is concentrated and enters or leaves the body. Traditionally, 365 acupoints were sited along the meridians but about 2,000 have now been identified and are depicted on modern acupuncture charts. These acupoints have a lower electrical resistance than the surrounding areas and can be pinpointed with great accuracy using a simple, hand-held device that measures electrical potential across the skin's surface.

The flow of *qi* depends on two opposite but complementary forces, *yin* and *yang*, a balance between which is necessary for well-being. This balance is easily disrupted by factors such as poor diet, stress, emotional distress, and spiritual neglect. Symptoms of illness are believed to be the result of blockages of energy along the meridians. Complementary therapies such as shiatsu, acupuncture, and acupressure are designed to stimulate acupoints, encouraging energy to enter or leave the body at these points, thus achieving balance and restoring harmony.

PRANA

In Ayurvedic medicine, *prana* is the dynamic energy or life force, similar to *qi*. We receive *prana* from three sources: the sun, the air, and the earth. Solar *prana* is absorbed during sunbathing or by drinking water that has been exposed

The theory of meridians envisages channels along which energy flows and acupoints are located.

to the sun; earth *prana* enters the body through the soles of the feet, while ozone *prana* is absorbed from the air during slow, deep breathing as part of relaxation or meditation.

The seat of *prana* is in the head, where it finds expression in the flow of intelligence and the control of the biological functions of two other, subtle essences known as *ojas* and *tejas*. Communication between body cells is known as pranic intelligence and is necessary for optimum function and coordination of tissues, organs, and body systems. If the flow of pranic energy is blocked, cellular chaos results, with the possible development of pain, illness, and even cancer. You can have too much *prana*, which may give rise to symptoms similar to those caused by stress (for example, disconnection, anxiety, fear, tremor, nausea, or diarrhea), or you can be deficient in *prana* energy, resulting in a lack of energy accompanied by lethargy, heaviness, depression, and hopelessness. A good diet, generally healthy lifestyle, adequate amounts of exercise, and supplements of herbal remedies are used to promote a balanced *prana*.

Prana absorbed from the sun, air, and earth is circulated around the body via energy centers known as *chakras*.

CHAKRAS

Chakras are life-energy distribution centers. There are seven situated down the middle – from the top of the head to the bottom of the trunk – of what is known as the subtle body, through which life energy flows. Each *chakra* produces energy for, or distributes it to, particular parts of the body. According to ancient yogic beliefs, breathing techniques, meditation, and yoga postures are supposed to encourage a type of energy known as *kundalini* to move from the lowest *chakra* to the highest, promoting spirituality, awareness, and divine knowledge. A blockage along an energy channel or in an underactive or overactive *chakra* results in pranic depletion or congestion.

Each *chakra* is associated with a particular color and is believed to have certain attributes (*see below*).

AURAS

Some people believe that everybody is surrounded by an aura of energy consisting of electromagnetic particles radiating from their body. Eastern philosophies believed that the aura energy emanates from the *hara*, situated just below the navel.

The human aura is believed to have seven layers, each relating to one of the seven *chakras*. The inner layer, closest to the skin, relates to health, while the outer layer is the spiritual layer. The *chakras* act as gateways between the aura and the body's energy distribution channels.

An aura is believed to consist of a series of colors that merge into one another and change from moment to moment. One is often dominant. When an aura is photographed (*see below*), it shows that aura at one particular moment. If another image is taken a few hours later,

CHAKRAS AND THEIR ATTRIBUTES

Chakra	Color	Attributes
Crown *chakra*	VIOLET	Deeply calming and relaxing; relieves insomnia, headache, stress, anxiety, and fear
Brow *chakra*	INDIGO	Strengthens intuition and heightens awareness; calming and relaxing
Throat *chakra*	BLUE	Encourages self-expression
Heart *chakra*	GREEN	Encourages inner peace, self-acceptance, and love; boosts immunity; balances hormones
Solar plexus *chakra*	YELLOW	Strengthens vitality and releases repressed emotions
Sacral *chakra*	ORANGE	Activates emotions and encourages openness and release; used to treat all urinary and genital problems
Root *chakra*	RED	Calming, reduces stress and tension; strengthens the spine and legs

Each *chakra* is also associated with a particular crystal that may be used to help boost energy levels at the sites of the *chakras* (*see also page 95*).

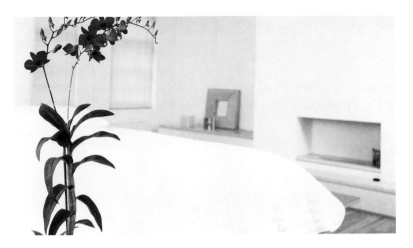

subtle differences will be apparent. A few days later, another image might be different still, since energy states are constantly changing. People with high energy levels may have an aura that stretches out three feet or more beyond their body, while those with depleted energy reserves may have an aura only a few inches wide.

DETECTING AURAS

Some people claim to be able to sense the aura of another person as vibrations, while others see colored lights. Auras can apparently be captured on film using techniques such as aura energy photography and Kirlian photography. The latter is a diagnostic technique that analyzes the body's electromagnetic field. An image is produced by placing parts of the body – usually hands or feet – on a photographic plate that emits a high-voltage, high-frequency electric signal. The interaction between this signal and the body's energy field is captured on film as an interference pattern. The shape and intensity of the image

Feng shui is the Chinese art of arranging your surroundings in accordance with universal energy to make an auspicious living space.

relates to your aura, and can reveal an energy imbalance between one side of the body and the other, for example, which is indicative of ill-health. These energy images can be related to acupuncture meridians.

You can detect your own energy aura by vigorously rubbing your hands together for a minute or so, then slowly separating them slightly and pushing them together again a few times. You should feel a slight force between your palms. You can strengthen this aura by holding a rock crystal while meditating. The energy of the crystal mingles with the aura energy of the person holding it (*see also page 95*).

COSMIC ENERGY

How we relate to energy on a larger scale can affect levels in our bodies, some believe. Energy fields in the environment created by natural phenomena such as the Earth's geology or the flow of underground water or man-made features such as power lines may affect health and cause what is know as geopathic stress. The Chinese practice of feng shui recommends arranging your environment in accordance with the forces of the universe. This entails assessing the flow of energy within your home (or place of work).

BIOELECTROMAGNETISM

Ancient philosophies about energy were based on an awareness that the human body generates its own electromagnetic field. Science now confirms that it does. The field arises from electrically charged particles (ions) that are dissolved in the fluid bathing all living cells. The membrane surrounding each cell

The body's electromagnetic energy field is said to be detectable as bands of colour radiating outwards and indicating your state of health.

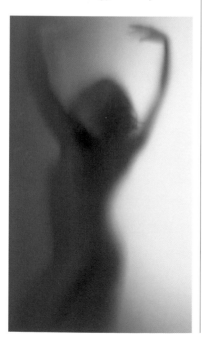

contains microscopic pores through which ions can flow into or out of each cell. Some pores have a pump action that enables them to move ions across a cell membrane so that they become concentrated on one side of the membrane or the other. One of the most important of these is the sodium-potassium pump.

This forces sodium ions out of body cells into the extracellular fluid surrounding them in exchange for potassium ions, which are forced into cells from the extracellular fluid. (Sodium is the main positively charged ion found in extracellular fluid while potassium is the main positively charged ion present inside the cells themselves.) The sodium-potassium pump transfers three positively charged sodium ions out of a cell in exchange for two positively charged potassium ions passing into the cell. In nerve cells the membrane electrical potential averages about -70 millivolts (mV), while the potential of other cells ranges from -9 mV to -100 mV.

This membrane potential of human body cells is important for the transmission of information along nerve fibers; for the passing of information from one cell to another; and for the contraction of muscle cells, including those of the heart creating a heartbeat.

MAGNETIC EFFECTS

Whenever an electric current flows or an electric field changes, it creates a magnetic field. The movement of electrically charged ions in and out of cells is the main source of the

THE CONCENTRATION OF IONS AROUND A SPINAL NERVE

ION	Concentration inside cell	Concentration outside cell
Sodium (Na+)	15 mmol/l	150 mmol/l
Potassium (K+)	150 mmol/l	5.5 mmol/l
Chloride (Cl-)	9 mmol/l	125 mmol/l

Resting membrane potential is -70 mV

body's electrical and magnetic fields. The generation and maintenance of this bioelectromagnetic energy field uses the greatest amount of energy of all human metabolic processes. On average, it accounts for 33 percent of the energy used by cells in general and 70 percent of energy expended by nerve cells (neurons).

THEORY AND PRACTICE

Many complementary treatments are based on the idea that the body's life energy travels along channels known as meridians. These can be compared to the flow patterns that exist in a magnetic field. If you are healthy, energy is flowing along its channels in a balanced way, but ill-health may result from interruptions or blockages in energy flow.

The body's electromagnetic field may be what is detected as life energy through acupoints on the surface of the skin. A technique that attempts to correct imbalances in the distribution of the body's electromagnetic energy is known as bioelectromagnetic therapy.

Rare-earth magnets made from an alloy of neodymium, iron, and boron are coated with purified zinc and surrounded with tiny copper spheres. These are attached to adhesive patches, which are applied to acupuncture points on the skin and are left undisturbed for five to seven days. This technique is used to relieve pain and stiffness associated with conditions such as arthritis, rheumatism, headaches or menstrual pain, and acts on nerve and muscle cells to relieve pain, relax tension, and improve circulation. It can also be applied to improve immunity and energy levels, relieving conditions such as insomnia and lack of energy.

BIOELECTROMAGNETISM AND HEALTH

Most illnesses affect the bioenergetic functions of cells, for example:

- The exchange of ions across cell membranes is altered by inflammation.
- Electrical transmission along nerves is increased when pain is perceived.
- Damaged body cells may leak potassium ions, producing a slow, steady electric current as much as 50 mV.
- Sudden electric fluxes occur when a cell dies and releases a burst of potassium ions.
- Changes in the composition of blood, other body fluids, and salt balance affect the nature of the body's electromagnetic field.

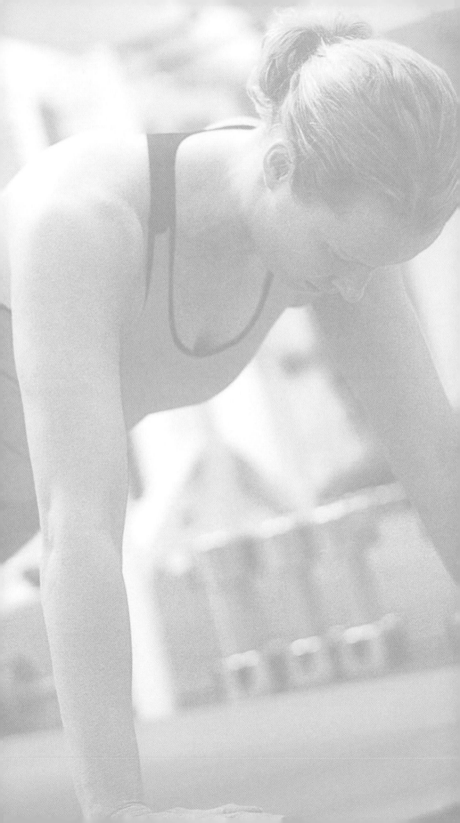

Boosting Energy

Improving low levels of physical, mental, and sexual energy may involve packing your diet with energy superfoods, trying nutritional supplements and herbal remedies, devising an exercise program that suits your physical needs and lifestyle, and employing spiritually therapeutic techniques to focus your mind and improve your mental and emotional well-being. All can be combined in an energy-boosting package.

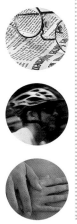

HOW MUCH ENERGY DO YOU HAVE?

Everyone has different amounts of energy at different times of the day, the week, or the month. If you feel that your energy levels are not what they should be, ask yourself a few basic questions to pinpoint the problems.

ASSESSING ENERGY LEVELS

Answer the following questions, responding fairly spontaneously and without giving them too much thought. Score two points for every "yes" answer, zero for a "no." Add up the points and analyze the results by turning to page 24.

If you decide that you would benefit from following an energy-boosting program such as those outlined on pages 112–23, ask yourself these questions again after you have implemented the program of your choice to see if your energy levels appear to have improved.

PHYSICAL ENERGY
Over the last couple of weeks, have you:

1	Needed less sleep than usual?		**6**	Been less stressed than usual?
2	Felt refreshed on waking?		**7**	Felt full of vitality?
3	Found it easy to get out of bed?		**8**	Had lots of energy for everyday tasks?
4	Felt youthful and rejuvenated?		**9**	Felt ready for a night on the town after work?
5	Enjoyed brisk physical activity?		**10**	Bounced through the day rather than dragging your heels?

Physical score: /20

MENTAL ENERGY
Over the last couple of weeks, have you:

11 Found it easy to concentrate?

16 Felt sociable and ready to meet new people?

12 Been able to remember things easily?

17 Been able to get more out of life?

13 Developed new interests?

18 Shown enthusiasm for new activities?

14 Felt creative at home or work?

19 Coped with extra pressure at home or work?

15 Been productive at home or work?

20 Felt in control of your emotions?

Mental score: /20

SEXUAL ENERGY
Over the last couple of weeks, have you:

21 Been aware of sensory enjoyment?

26 Become sexually aroused easily?

22 Had thoughts about sex several times a day?

27 Felt like initiating sex?

23 Wanted to make love at least once a week?

28 Reached sexual climax easily?

24 Planned a romantic occasion?

29 Made love more than once during lovemaking?

25 Talked about love or sex with a friend or partner?

30 Thought about starting a family or having more children?

Sexual score: /20

SCORE
Physical energy

0–9
Your physical energy levels are significantly depleted and you would benefit greatly from following an energy-boosting program.

10–15
Your physical energy levels are acceptable, but you may feel drained after a particularly stressful event or if you have had less sleep than usual. An energy-boosting program should be able to improve your vitality.

16–20
You appear to have plenty of zest for life. Maintain this optimum state by examining your diet and lifestyle and perhaps taking supplements.

SCORE
Mental energy

0–9
You would benefit greatly from following an energy-boosting program. You might also benefit from going on vacation and recharging your batteries.

10–15
Your mental energy levels are acceptable, but it may sometimes be hard to concentrate, remember things, or cope with new pressures. An energy-boosting program will help you meet life's challenges more readily.

16–20
You certainly seem to have plenty of mental energy, and appear more than capable of dealing with anything life may throw at you.

SCORE
Sexual energy

0–9
Your sexual energy levels are depleted and you should consider an energy-boosting program and an adaptogen supplement such as ginseng.

10–15
Your sexual energy levels are normal, but you may find you do not feel like having sex if you are tired and drained. Following an energy-boosting program will give your sexual energy levels a welcome boost.

16–20
You appear to have a healthy level of sexual energy, which suggests that love and sex are subjects never far from your thoughts.

NEED TO SEE A DOCTOR?

Sometimes a lack of energy can be indicative of a medical condition that may need investigation and treatment. If you feel your energy levels are persistently or seriously low, consult your doctor in case exploratory tests are necessary.

AILMENTS WITH LACK OF ENERGY AS A SYMPTOM

- Anemia – especially iron-deficiency anemia
- Underactive thyroid (hypothyroidism)
- Overactive thyroid (hyperthyroidism)
- Depression
- Seasonal Affective Disorder (SAD)
- Side effects of medication
- Poorly controlled diabetes
- Uncontrolled high blood pressure
- Irregular heartbeat
- Heart failure (causing fluid retention)
- Infection – especially mononucleosis or long-term grumbling infections
- Chronic inflammatory disease (for example, rheumatoid arthritis)
- Autoimmune disorder (for example, Systemic Lupus Erythematosus/SLE)
- Disease of any organ system (such as the lungs, kidneys, or liver)
- Chronic fatigue syndrome (Myalgic Encephalomyelitis/ME)
- Serious illness such as cancer

ENERGY FOODS

ALL THE ENERGY PRODUCED BY THE
BODY IS ULTIMATELY DERIVED FROM
FOOD. SOME FOODS ARE EXCEPTIONALLY
GOOD AT BOOSTING ENERGY, PROVIDING
CARBOHYDRATE, PROTEIN, OR FATTY
ACIDS AS FUEL AS WELL AS IMPORTANT
VITAMINS, MINERALS, AND TRACE
ELEMENTS. IT IS ADVISABLE TO
CONCENTRATE ON EATING FOODS
THAT PEP YOU UP AND TO AVOID THOSE
THAT HAVE THE OPPOSITE EFFECT.

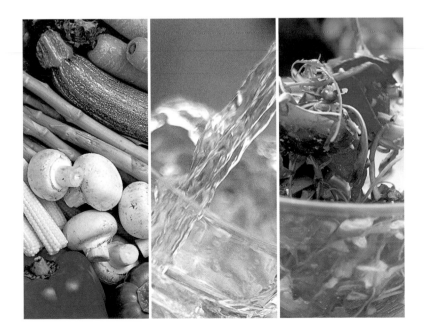

THE ENERGY IN FOOD

The expression "you are what you eat" is increasingly shown to be true. Every body cell is ultimately derived from food, which provides all the components and energy we need for optimum health and energy levels.

ENERGY COMPONENTS

The energy in food comes from fats, carbohydrates, and proteins. Fats provide more than twice as many calories, gram for gram, as proteins or carbohydrates. Carbohydrates are made up of simple sugars (for example, glucose) which raise blood sugar levels quickly, providing a short-term energy boost. Complex carbohydrates (such as starch) are made up of chains of simple sugars that must be broken down before they can be used. They thus provide a more sustained supply of energy.

THE BEST CARBOHYDRATES

Eating too many simple sugars (such as potatoes) is not advisable. They trigger release of insulin, produced to regulate blood sugar levels, which then tend to fall quickly. You should aim to obtain at least half your energy from complex carbohydrates (such as green vegetables and legumes) to ensure sustained energy levels. The rate at which food raises blood sugar levels is identified by its glycemic index (GI). It is best to eat foods with a low to moderate GI or combine high- with low-GI-foods.

GLYCEMIC INDEX OF COMMON FOODS

Food	GI	Food	GI
Glucose	100	Whole-wheat pasta	42
Baked potatoes	98	Baked beans	40
Parsnips	97	Oranges	40
Carrots	92	Apples	39
Cornflakes	84	Ice-cream	36
Brown rice	82	Milk	32
Whole-wheat bread	72	Butter	<30
Chocolate bar	68	Cheese	<30
Cream of wheat	66	Eggs	<30
Muesli	66	Fish	<30
Raisins	64	Seafood	<30
Bananas	62	Meat	<30
Chocolate cookie	59	Green vegetables	<30
Bran Chex	58	Plums	<30
Oatmeal	54	Grapefruit	<30
Potato chips	51	Peanuts	<30
Grapes	44	Legumes	<30

FOOD PRODUCTION TODAY

The qualities of food that we have come to expect are often achieved at the expense of flavor and nutrient content, and with the help of agrochemicals such as pesticides, fertilizers, weedkillers, fumigants, and growth promoters and retardants.

THE RISK FROM CHEMICALS

Chemicals are applied to crops throughout the growing cycle. They do not just lie on the surface but permeate the skin and flesh. These chemicals are supposed to be safe, but the full effects of many of them on human energy levels and long-term health are still not fully understood. There is evidence that many chemicals are not used correctly, so food might contain dangerous amounts of some and traces of others that are prohibited.

A lot of food is produced using methods that enhance its color and make items of a uniform size so that it looks appealing for as long as possible.

GOING ORGANIC

Increasing numbers of people are choosing to eat organic foods with minimal processing. Organic farming practices involve sustainable methods that work with, not against, nature and avoid the use of artificial fertilizers and pesticides, antibiotics, genetic manipulation, hormones, or irridation. Instead, farmers use traditional methods of pest control, crop rotation, growing green manure crops (such as clover) and carefully timing of the sowing of crops. As a result, organic foods may be more nutritious and may taste better. They are also more likely to improve energy levels.

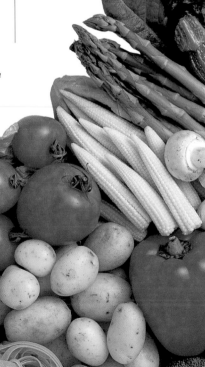

FOODS TO PEP YOU UP

Include certain types of food in your diet to ensure a natural energy boost. The foods that have the greatest potential for boosting your energy are very often the same as those foods recommended for maintaining general good health.

GOOD FOODS

- Whole-grain cereals, such as oats, rice, pasta, bread, and breakfast cereals
- Whole-wheat breads – especially those with added nuts and seeds
- Root vegetables, such as carrots, parsnips, turnips, rutabagas, and potatoes
- Cruciferous plants, for example broccoli, cabbage, and Chinese cabbage
- Legumes, such as lentils, kidney beans, and soybeans
- Fresh fruit, for example avocados, bananas, melon, plums, grapes, oranges, and pineapple
- Ready-to-eat, semidried fruit, such as apricots, dates, figs, and prunes
- Oily fish
- Virgin olive oil
- Nuts – especially walnuts – and seeds
- Honey (in moderation)

FRUIT FOR ENERGY

Fresh fruit provides fruit sugars for an instant yet healthy energy boost plus complex carbohydrates for a more prolonged energy burst. The

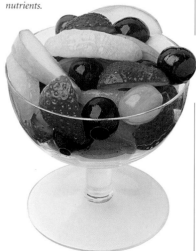

Fruit is best eaten raw or only lightly cooked to preserve as much goodness as possible. It provides water in addition to vitamins, minerals, and other nutrients.

latter ensure sugars are released gradually into the bloodstream to maintain the stable blood glucose levels needed for optimum energy production. In addition, fruit contains fiber – essential for healthy digestion – and a variety of beneficial vitamins, minerals and nonnutrient plant substances (phytochemicals). For example, fruit is rich in potassium, which is an important mineral for nerve and muscle function, and it contains bioflavonoids that have vital antioxidant, antiviral, and antibacterial actions.

Healthy eating guidelines usually recommend five or more servings of fruit or vegetables (not including potatoes) a day – and more if at all possible. Organically grown fruit is the best choice, since agrochemicals are widely suspected of damaging the body's immune system.

BREAKING YOUR FAST

At least one person in six does not eat breakfast regularly, even though this is the most important meal for restoring energy levels. Among the best foods for a "power" breakfast are unsweetened cereal, fruit, and lowfat or nonfat milk.

For maximum energy, spread your consumption of food evenly throughout the day. It is better to eat three medium-sized meals than several snacks and a huge supper.

Between-meal snacks used to be frowned on, but they can help to boost metabolic rates.

FOODS THAT DRAG YOU DOWN

Eating too many of the wrong kinds of food will quickly leave you feeling bloated and slowed-down. Fatty foods for breakfast may reduce your concentration all morning. If you also eat a fatty lunch, you will function below par all day.

NOT-SO-GOOD FOODS

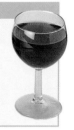

+ Fatty, sugary snacks, such as doughnuts or pastries
+ Fatty, salty snacks such as potato chips or pepperoni pizza
+ Cakes, cookies, and confectionery
+ Red meat
+ Alcohol – have no more than one glass of wine, preferably red, a day
+ Products containing caffeine

"GOOD" AND "BAD" FATS

Fats are the richest dietary source of energy but, unfortunately, a lot of people eat too many "bad" fats (such as trans fats, which are found in hard margarines and many processed baked foods) and not enough "good" fats, which are found in oily fish, nuts, seeds, and olives. You should try to consume more of the healthy fats while reducing your overall fat intake. As well as boosting your energy levels, this will help you shift excess weight.

TIPS FOR HEALTHY EATING

+ Concentrate on obtaining healthy, essential fatty acids from nuts, seeds, whole grains, oily fish, olive oil, canola oil, evening primrose oil, and green leafy vegetables
+ Avoid obviously fatty foods
+ Use only lean cuts of meat and trim excess fat
+ Eat chicken in preference to fatty meats such as pork
+ Broil food rather than frying it to help fat drain away
+ Soak up excess fat from cooked foods using paper towel
+ Eat baked rather than roasted potatoes or french fries
+ Choose lowfat varieties of mayonnaise, salad dressing, cheese, milk, and yogurt
+ Reduce your intakes of margarine and processed foods

THE IMPORTANCE OF FLUIDS

Water makes up as much as 60 percent of your body weight. All metabolic processes and body systems depend on it – fluids are necessary to flush toxins and wastes through the kidneys, for example.

Most people would benefit from increasing their fluid intake. One of the consequences of dehydration is a loss of energy and tiredness. So try to drink at least three to four pints of fluid a day – and even more when you are exercising and during hot weather. Keep a bottle of water with you at all times and sip it frequently, or choose herbal and fruit teas or green tea as a delicious way of

Tea is one of the most popular drinks in the world and its health benefits are well documented: it contains antioxidants, for example.

maintaining your fluid intakes. Keep drinks containing a lot of caffeine to a minimum.

A HEALTHY CUP

Both green and black tea are made from the young leaves and leaf buds of *Camellia sinensis*. The black tea with which we are probably most familiar is made by crushing and fermenting freshly cut tea leaves before drying them. This allows natural enzymes in the tea leaves to produce the characteristic red-brown color and reduces the astringency. Green tea is made by steaming or drying fresh tea leaves immediately after cutting.

The type of antioxidants present in tea depends on how it is made. Green tea contains high levels of naturally occurring, powerful flavonoids known as catechins. These are lost during the fermentation process, but are converted into other types of flavonoid antioxidants that are themselves beneficial to health. Modern scientific research confirms the ancient Chinese belief in the health-giving properties of tea. Drinking four to five cups a day has been linked to lower blood cholesterol levels, lower blood pressure, and a reduced risk of coronary heart disease and stroke. It has also been shown to reduce the risk of some types of cancer developing. For people feeling tired or weary, many claim, there is nothing quite like a cup of tea for a healthy pick-me-up.

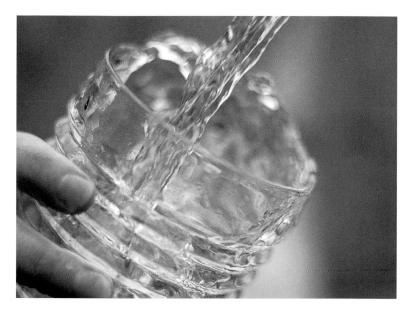

THE GREAT ENERGY DRAINER

Caffeine mimics the effects of stress on the body and increases levels of stress hormones such as epinephrine and cortisol in the blood stream. In addition, it does away with one of the body's natural safety valves by blocking the effects of a calming brain chemical known as adenosine. Adenosine has other actions, including storing and producing energy. Overall, adenosine helps to balance the body's response to stress. If its actions are blocked by excessive amounts of caffeine, you will succumb to the effects of stress more quickly and soon start to feel drained of energy.

People metabolize caffeine at different rates. Some metabolize it slowly and become irritable and jittery quickly, while others seem to consume huge quantities with no apparent ill-effects. A person weighing 155 pounds (70 kg) who

Try to drink about eight glasses of water a day. Water is continually being lost from the body and needs to be replenished.

drinks more than six caffeine-containing drinks – for example four cups of coffee and two cola drinks – a day is at risk of caffeine poisoning. (Tea does contain caffeine, but less than coffee.) This may manifest itself in symptoms such as restlessness, insomnia, headaches, anxiety, and fatigue. Smokers produce liver enzymes that encourage the breakdown of caffeine, and they flush it out of their bodies 50 percent faster than nonsmokers. Alcohol reduces the rate at which caffeine is cleared from the body, while hormonal methods of contraception may triple the time it stays in the body.

If you feel lacking in energy, it is advisable to cut right back on caffeine or, better still, eliminate it from your diet altogether.

WHOLE GRAINS

Excellent carbohydrate source ◆ High-fiber foods

◆ Reduce the risk of coronary heart disease

OATS

Cereals are cultivated grasses from which the grains are harvested and made into cereal products. Oats are nutritious cereals whose grains may be rolled, flaked, or ground to make oatmeal or flour.

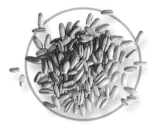

They are mainly eaten as porridge or as an ingredient in granola.

Oats are a particularly good source of complex carbohydrates, which help to sustain blood-sugar levels. They are good for maintaining a healthy weight as well as energy levels. Australian research found that athletes who followed an oat-based diet for three weeks showed a 4 percent increase in stamina.

Oats have a soothing effect on the nervous system, and oatstraw is a popular tonic for nervous exhaustion. Oats are also believed to help reduce cravings, and oatmeal or granola are good foods for people trying to quit

KEY BENEFITS

Oats contain more protein than any other cereal, are a good source of soluble fiber, and contain useful amounts of B-group vitamins. which are needed for producing energy. They also supply many minerals, including calcium, iron, and trace elements.

smoking, for example. Traditionally, oats have a reputation for boosting sexual energy levels, hence the popular saying about sowing your wild oats.

Finally, oatbran has been demonstrated to help reduce high levels of cholesterol in the blood and, if it is included regularly in the diet, helps to ease constipation.

Nutritional values per 100 g	
OATS	
Carbohydrate	66 g
Starch	65 g
Sugars	1 g
Protein	11 g
Fat	9 g
Energy	375 cal
Glycemic Index	medium

GRANOLA	
Carbohydrate	72 g
Starch	46 g
Sugars	26 g
Protein	10 g
Fat	6 g
Energy	363 cal
Glycemic Index	high

MAKING MUESLI

Energizing muesli provides an immediate as well as a sustained energy boost because it combines oats, a source of slow-energy-release carbohydrates, with dried fruits, which contain more instantly accessible simple sugars. Nuts and seeds add extra nutritional value, including essential fatty acids, while toasted wheatflakes and bran flakes provide crunch.

FRUIT, NUT & SEED MUESLI

4 oz (100 g) dried apricots, chopped

2 oz (50 g) each of rolled oats, toasted wheatflakes, rye flakes, barley flakes, bran buds or flakes, chopped dried dates, chopped dried figs, chopped walnuts, and pine nuts

1 oz (25 g) each of chopped brazil nuts, chopped filberts and poppy, sesame, sunflower, and pumpkin seeds

Mix alll the ingredients and store in an airtight container. Shake well before serving. Serve with milk, fromage frais, or yogurt, all lowfat.

BREAKFAST CEREALS

One of the main reasons why a cereal breakfast is so good for you is that it provides essential brain fuel, glucose, at a crucial time of the day – after a long, overnight fast. Most are made from corn, wheat, or bran.

There is plenty of evidence to support the idea that eating cereals at the beginning of the day will improve memory, the recall of new information, the ability to concentrate, and general mental ability.

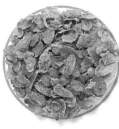

Schoolchildren who eat breakfast, including cereal, perform better than those who do not. They exhibit more extensive word power, a greater ability to absorb new information, improved problem-solving skills, and better physical endurance. Exam results may be influenced by whether students have eaten breakfast on the day they are tested. In one group of ten-year-olds, those who had eaten a carbohydrate-rich breakfast made fewer mistakes and worked quicker in a math test than those who had not.

In studies of healthy adults over the age of 60,

KEY BENEFITS

Unsweetened cereals are an excellent low-fat, high-carbohydrate source of energy. If eaten for breakfast, they improve both physical and mental performance and emotional stability throughout the day. Not only will you keep going for longer, you will be less likely to feel dispirited and you will not become stressed as easily as you will if you start the day with a less energizing breakfast.

it was found that those who ate a breakfast cereal regularly performed better in national adult reading tests (which are closely linked to intelligence quotient) than those who did not. Whether this is because intelligent people choose to eat breakfast cereals or because eating breakfast cereals improves intelligence is, however, open to debate.

Eating a breakfast that provides plenty of carbohydrate is also very necessary if you have a physically demanding job or are an athlete. This is particularly relevant for those who undertake prolonged exercise such as long-distance running, cycling, and triathlon events, and for those who play certain team sports.

Breakfast cereals that contain bran provide one of the best concentrations of dietary fiber: 2 oz (40 g) per 4 oz (100 g) cereal.

MOOD FOOD

There appears to be a complex link between what you eat for breakfast and your mood. The means by which carbohydrates affect mood may only occur when you wake up in the morning and not later on in the day. Cereals are a rich source of vitamin B_1 (thiamine) which has a beneficial effect on mood, making you feel more calm, agreeable, clear-headed, elated, and energetic. Those people who have low levels of thiamine are less likely to feel composed or self-confident and are more likely to suffer from emotional distress or depression than those with higher levels of this important vitamin.

Nutritional values per 100 g

BRAN FLAKES	
Carbohydrate	70 g
Starch	51 g
Sugars	19 g
Protein	10 g
Fat	2 g
Energy	318 cal
Glycemic Index	medium

CORNFLAKES	
Carbohydrate	86 g
Starch	78 g
Sugars	8 g
Protein	11 g
Fat	3 g
Energy	325 cal
Glycemic Index	high

WEETABIX	
Carbohydrate	76 g
Starch	71 g
Sugars	5 g
Protein	11 g
Fat	3 g
Energy	352 cal
Glycemic Index	high

BROWN RICE

Rice is a staple food for more than half the Earth's population, for whom it provides both energy and protein. Its nutritional value is greatly reduced, however, if it is milled to remove the bran, which provides fiber, B-group vitamins, minerals such as calcium, zinc, and magnesium as well as a delicious nutty flavor. The

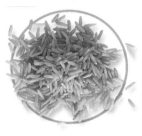

B-group vitamins are locked into the bran and only released into the grain when it is cooked. As a result, those who eat only white rice may be more at risk of the vitamin-B deficiency disease, beriberi, while those who eat brown rice or rice that was parboiled before milling, are not. Parboiled rice is often described as "quick rice."

The versatility of rice also makes it a valuable addition to the diet. It can be boiled, steamed, baked (in fluid such as milk), or fried. Traditional dishes around the world include paella, risotto, egg foo yong, kedgeree, and rice pudding. It can also be made into ricecakes using puffed rice. Wild rice is not a true rice but the grain of a North American wild grass. It is often added to basmati rice for a black-and-white effect.

Nutritional values per 100 g BROWN RICE	
Carbohydrate	32 g
Starch	31 g
Sugars	1 g
Protein	3 g
Fat	1 g
Energy	141 cal
Glycemic Index	high

WHOLE-WHEAT PASTA

Pasta is an Italian staple made from high-protein durum wheat flour or semolina and water.

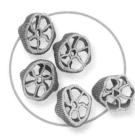

Ingredients such as eggs, spinach, herbs, garlic, tomatoes, beets, or even squid ink may be added to pasta for variety of both color and flavour.

Whole-wheat pasta is a good source of B-group vitamins – especially B_1,

or thiamin – which are important in energy-generating processes.

Pasta has a reputation for being fattening among many people watching their weight, but this is only the case if it is served with lots of butter, cheese, or cream-based sauce. If served the Italian way, that is, very simply with a minimum amount of sauce, it is useful as part of a diet for maintaining a healthy weight. Pasta combines particularly well with vegetarian sauces that are based on combinations of olive oil, garlic, tomatoes, and a variety of herbs.

Traditionally, wheat has been used in Eastern medicine to promote calm and composure, to focus the mind, and to encourage restful sleep.

Nutritional values per 100 g WHOLE-WHEAT PASTA	
Carbohydrate	23 g
Starch	22 g
Sugars	1 g
Protein	5 g
Fat	1 g
Energy	113 cal
Glycemic Index	medium

BREAD

Bread is a dietary staple. All types of whole-grain bread are good energy sources and can be eaten at all meals. Bread is such a good carbohydrate supply that most healthy eating guidelines suggest at least five slices a day.

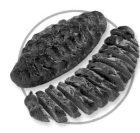

Sandwiches and rolls are the most widely eaten healthy snacks. Like pasta, bread has a reputation for being fattening, but it is the fillings that tend to be responsible rather than the bread itself.

KEY BENEFITS

Whole-grain bread is a good source of energy in the form of complex carbohydrate, which releases glucose gradually into the bloodstream. It is also a good source of fiber, B-group vitamins, and essential minerals as well as trace elements.

Bread made from brown (whole-wheat) flour instead of white (refined) flour supplies more fiber. Foods containing 3 g of fiber per 100 g or more are considered high-fiber, and brown bread typically provides 6 g. It is also a rich source of vitamins, especially the B-group, which are important in the metabolic processes that generate energy, minerals – especially iron and calcium – and trace elements. It also has a delicious nutty flavor. The flour used to make brown and white bread is enhanced by law by the addition of iron, thiamin, riboflavin, and niacin. The only flour that does not need to be enriched is whole-wheat.

Nutritional values per 100 g	
WHOLE-WHEAT BREAD	
Carbohydrate	44 g
Starch	40 g
Sugars	2 g
Protein	9 g
Fat	2 g
Energy	218 cal
Glycemic Index	high

WHOLE-GRAIN BREAD	
Carbohydrate	46 g
Starch	44 g
Sugars	2 g
Protein	9 g
Fat	3 g
Energy	235 cal
Glycemic Index	high

HEALTHY VARIETY

Many kinds of breads are now widely available, and bread machines encourage people to make their own bread. Nuts, seeds, herbs, soyflour, garlic, and dried fruit may be added for flavor, texture, and extra nutrients.

Ciabatta bread is made with all-purpose or whole-wheat flour to which olive oil is added.
Focaccia is made from dough flavored with olive oil, salt, herbs, and garlic and baked in a flat round pan similar to a pizza base.
Pita bread is flat and made from all-purpose or whole-wheat flour. It is split open to reveal a pocket that can be easily stuffed.
Pumpernickel is a heavy, dark brown rye bread that is steamed as well as baked to produce a moist texture and rich flavor.
Rye bread is made with rye or wheat and rye flour to produce a heavy, dense, dark-colored loaf that has a slightly sour flavor.

FLOUR POWER

The flour that is used to make bread largely determines its type.

Brown bread is made from stone-ground flour from which some of the bran has been removed.
Whole-wheat bread is made from whole-wheat flour or white flour that has added bran and wheat germ.
White bread is made from flour that is steel-ground, stripping away the wheat germ, destroying nutrients.
High-fiber white bread is made with all-purpose flour enriched with added rice-bran or soy-hull fiber.
Soy and linseed flour bread is rich in beneficial plant estrogens, and may help reduce unpleasant menopausal symptoms, such as fatigue, hot flashes, and night sweats.

ROOT VEGETABLES

Provide vitamins and important plant nutrients

◆ Lowfat energy foods ◆ Good source of fiber

JERUSALEM ARTICHOKES

Jerusalem artichokes are tubers derived from the American sunflower. Selective breeding has resulted in smoother tubers that are easier to clean and prepare and that look better. Jerusalem

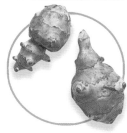

artichokes can be eaten boiled, with or without a sauce; cut in half, brushed with olive oil, and broiled; or made into soup.

A healthy digestion is important for maintaining

KEY BENEFITS

This vegetable is a good carbohydrate source. As the vegetable matures, starches are converted into digestible sugars so it becomes sweeter and its energy potential increases. Artichokes contain an enzyme, inulase, and a complex sugar, inulin, which aids digestion. Inulin and inulase help to stabilize glucose levels.

optimum energy levels, and Jerusalem artichokes are a rich source of fructo-oligosaccharides (FOS). These have what is known as a prebiotic action in the body. Prebiotics encourage the growth of "friendly" digestive bacteria in the gut such as *Lactobacilli*, which improve digestion and reduce the risk of intestinal ailments such as gastroenteritis developing.

Jerusalem artichokes are a good source of the mineral potassium and they also contain useful amounts of calcium, magnesium, and iron.

Nutritional values per 100 g JERUSALEM ARTICHOKES	
Carbohydrate	11 g
Starch	<1 g
Sugars	11 g
Protein	2 g
Fat	<1 g
Energy	41 cal
Glycemic Index	low

CARROTS

The Ancient Greeks believed that all parts of the carrot were an aphrodisiac. They would eat the seeds, root, and foliage before an orgy to boost their sexual energy.

Although they are only 8 percent carbohydrate, carrots are a useful source of fiber, potassium, and other minerals used in

KEY BENEFITS

Carrots are a very rich source of carotenoids – the yellow-orange pigments that give the vegetables their color. These are important antioxidants, which help protect against coronary artery disease and several cancers.

energy production. The carotenoids they contain are very important since alpha- and beta-carotene can be converted by the body into vitamin A. Carotenoids also protect

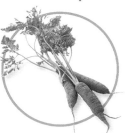

the part of the eye's retina that is responsible for fine vision, so the old saying that eating carrots helps you see in the dark has a foundation in reality.

Nutritional values per 100 g CARROTS	
Carbohydrate	8 g
Starch	0 g
Sugars	8 g
Protein	<1 g
Fat	<1 g
Energy	35 cal
Glycemic Index	high

POTATOES

Probably the best-loved root vegetable, the potato is one of the main starchy staple foods. Like other high-carbohydrate foods, they have a reputation for being fattening, but it is usually the way they are cooked or other

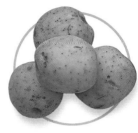

ingredients they are served with that are responsible. A baked potato makes an excellent, filling, energy-rich snack. For optimum health, eat potatoes simply boiled in their skins, mashed, baked in their skins, or added to stews, casseroles, or soups. Roasting them in a little oil (such as olive) means that less fat is absorbed into the potato's flesh than during deep frying.

Potatoes contain hydroxycinnamic acids,

which are antioxidants, as well as being a source of vitamins B and C, iron, and potassium. Most of these nutrients are found just beneath the potato's skin, so eating scrubbed, unpeeled potatoes is much better for boosting energy levels and general health than eating them peeled. The vitamin-C content of potatoes starts to decrease as soon as they are harvested, so they should also be consumed as fresh as possible.

Avoid eating sprouted or green potatoes, which contain the toxic alkaloids chaconine and solanine. These can cause vomiting and diarrhea, migraines, or drowsiness. They may also be harmful to a fetus during pregnancy.

Nutritional values per 100 g	
POTATOES	
Carbohydrate	17 g
Starch	16 g
Sugars	1 g
Protein	2 g
Fat	<1 g
Energy	75 cal
Glycemic Index	high

SWEET POTATOES

Sweet potatoes – also sometimes known as yams – are eaten in a similar way to ordinary potatoes. There are two kinds – the moist, orange-fleshed tubers and a drier, creamy-fleshed version.

A good source of the main dietary antioxidants (carotenoids and vitamins C and E), sweet potatoes are a valuable addition to the diet. Carotenoids help reduce the risk of age-

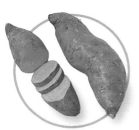

related degeneration of the retina in which fine vision is lost. Carotenoids also help to protect the skin from sun damage and may protect against inflammatory conditions such as arthritis and some forms of cancer.

Sweet potatoes also contain useful amounts of potassium, magnesium, vitamin C, vitamin E, and fiber, plus small amounts of minerals important for energy production.

A relation of the sweet potato, the Mexican wild yam, contains hormonal building blocks with an action like progesterone. These are used as a basis for some alternatives to estrogen-based HRT.

Nutritional values per 100 g	
SWEET POTATOES	
Carbohydrate	21 g
Starch	15 g
Sugars	6 g
Protein	1 g
Fat	<1 g
Energy	87 cal
Glycemic Index	high

GREEN VEGETABLES

Contain vitamins, minerals for energy production, and
protective plant nutrients ◆ High-fiber, lowfat food

BROCCOLI

This is one of the most
beneficial green vegetables
because of its protective
phytonutrients. Broccoli
should only be steamed
or boiled briefly to help

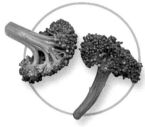

preserve its beneficial
components, and it can
be eaten raw in salads for
optimum nutrition.
Broccoli sprouts, a rich
source of phytochemicals,
are delicious raw.

Broccoli contains
calcium as well as useful
amounts of magnesium,
vital for producing energy
and for muscle function
and nerve conduction. It
also contains weak plant
estrogens, which are
converted by intestinal
bacteria into hormone-
like substances, especially
if the diet is rich in fiber.
Broccoli also contains
vitamin C, folic acid, iron,
potassium, carotenoids,
and indole-3-carbinol, a
substance needed by the
body to metabolize sex
hormones efficiently.

Nutritional values per 100 g
BROCCOLI

Carbohydrate	2 g
Starch	<1 g
Sugars	2 g
Protein	4 g
Fat	1 g
Energy	33 cal
Glycemic Index	low

CABBAGE

There is a large variety of
cabbage, which includes
collard greens, red and
white cabbage, and Savoy.
Cabbage juice may be
given to convalescents

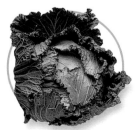

since it reduces inflam-
mation. As sauerkraut,
it encourages a healthy
balance of intestinal
bacteria.

Cabbage is a good
source of vitamins B_1, C,
and E, folate, carotenes,
and S-methylmethionine,
a substance that helps
relieve stomach ulcers.

Members of the
cabbage family (cabbage,
cauliflower, spinach,
Brussels sprouts, broccoli,
rutabagas, and turnips)
do contain substances
that interfere with the
action of iodine. You need
to absorb plenty of iodine
if you are lacking energy,
so eat these vegetables
only in moderation if
you are trying to boost
your energy levels.

KEY BENEFITS

Broccoli contributes to
long-term vitality by
helping to protect the
body against cancer. It
does this by means of
sulforaphane, an
antioxidant that has
powerful anticancer
properties, especially
against tumors of the
digestive tract, lungs,
and prostate gland. It
works by activating the
body's own detoxifying
enzyme systems.

KEY BENEFITS

From an energy point
of view, cabbage is
four percent sugar. It is
a good source of folate,
needed for red blood-
cell production, and
phytochemicals that
protect against cancer.

Nutritional values per 100 g
CABBAGE

Carbohydrate	2 g
Starch	<1 g
Sugars	3 g
Protein	3 g
Fat	1 g
Energy	33 cal
Glycemic Index	low

SPINACH

Popeye's favorite energy-boosting food contains lots of carotenoids and folate as well as useful amounts of magnesium, potassium, calcium, iron, and vitamins C and E.

Folate and folic acid (a synthetic form of folate),

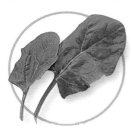

help reduce the risk of a woman conceiving a child with certain congenital abnormalities. A daily intake of 200 mcg of dietary folate plus 400 mcg of supplements and an increased intake of foods fortified with folic acid is recommended for women planning to conceive and for at least

KEY BENEFITS

Spinach is one of the richest dietary sources of folate, which is required for a number of metabolic reactions including protein and sugar metabolism. If folate is in short supply, a form of anemia may develop that quickly leads to tiredness and a lack of energy. In a study of 60 people who had chronic fatigue syndrome, at least 50 percent of them had low levels of folate.

the first three months of pregnancy. Folate is also believed to protect against coronary heart disease by helping to reduce raised blood levels of an amino acid called homocysteine.

Folate plays a role in chromosome replication during cell division so dietary sources may protect against cancer.

Prolonged boiling removes much of the folate content of green leafy vegetables, however, so they are best steamed. Folate is also destroyed by exposure to light and air.

Nutritional values per 100 g SPINACH	
Carbohydrate	2 g
Starch	<1 g
Sugars	2 g
Protein	3 g
Fat	1 g
Energy	25 cal
Glycemic Index	low

CURLY KALE

Like spinach, this is a rich source of folate, vitamin C, and carotenoids. It also contains useful amounts of potassium, calcium,

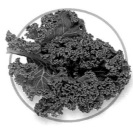

magnesium, iron, and manganese as well as selenium if it is grown in soils rich in this mineral.

Both curly kale and spinach are excellent sources of calcium, which

KEY BENEFITS

From an energy point of view, curly kale is low in carbohydrate, but its dietary value comes from a relatively high iron content (needed for oxygen-carrying purposes), making it important for those who do not eat red meat. The iron present in spinach, curly kale, and other vegetables is in the nonhaem form. This is not as well absorbed as the haem form found in meats. Nevertheless, the vitamin-C content of dark green leafy vegetables improves the iron's absorption.

is very important for strong bones and teeth as well as for muscle contraction and nerve-impulse conduction. These vegetables have the additional benefits of protecting against age-related degeneration of the retina – a common cause of reduced vision in older people – by virtue of the carotenoids (such as lutein) they contain. The color of these yellow-orange pigments is concealed by the high level of chlorophyll present in these plants.

Nutritional values per 100 g CURLY KALE	
Carbohydrate	1 g
Starch	<1 g
Sugars	1 g
Protein	3 g
Fat	2 g
Energy	33 cal
Glycemic Index	low

LEGUMES

Provide protective plant nutrients ◆ Protein source

◆ Stabilize blood-sugar levels ◆ Useful source of minerals

CHICKPEAS

Chickpeas can be added to soups, casseroles, and stews, eaten whole as a vegetable accompaniment, or mashed and combined with lemon juice, olive oil, and sesame seed puree (tahini) to make houmus.

They provide protein but, like most legumes, are considered a second-

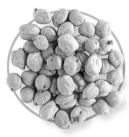

class protein source since some important amino acids are missing. They are best combined with other plant foods and whole grains such as rice and bread to balance amino-acid intakes.

Chickpeas are a good source of estrogen-like

KEY BENEFITS

Chickpeas provide carbohydrate that is slowly digested and absorbed, giving you a prolonged energy boost. They are also an important source of vitamins, minerals, and phytonutrients.

isoflavones. These plant hormones help rectify hormonal imbalances that are a common cause of reduced physical, mental, and sexual energy. Eating more isoflavonoid-rich foods such as chickpeas can therefore provide you with an energy boost.

Chickpeas also supply potassium, calcium, magnesium, and folate. They have useful amounts of iron, zinc, manganese, selenium, vitamin E, and B-group vitamins.

Nutritional values per 100 g	
CHICKPEAS (COOKED)	
Carbohydrate	18 g
Starch	17 g
Sugars	1 g
Protein	8 g
Fat	2 g
Energy	121 cal
Glycemic Index	low

SOYBEANS

Soybeans may be red, black, or white, and are added to many products – from bread to granola bars – because of their immense health benefits.

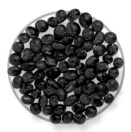

KEY BENEFITS

Soybeans are a high-class source of protein, comparable to meat in their amino-acid content. They also provide a significant amount of energy in the form of fat and carbohydrate. Their starches are digested slowly, providing a steady glucose supply.

Soybeans and soy products, such as tofu, miso, soy milk, and soy sauce, contribute to long-term vitality. They are rich sources of estrogen-like plant hormones that protect against reduced-energy states linked to hormonal imbalance such as that occurring during menopause. Just 60 g a day may be enough.

Based on the findings of more than 50 studies, the US Food and Drug Administration have authorized the claim that "a diet low in saturated fat and cholesterol, and which includes 25 g soy protein a day, can reduce the risk of coronary heart disease significantly." In addition, isoflavonoids protect against cancer.

Soybeans also supply many important minerals, trace elements, folate, and B-group vitamins.

Nutritional values per 100 g SOYBEANS (COOKED)	
Carbohydrate	5 g
Starch	2 g
Sugars	3 g
Protein	14 g
Fat	7 g
Energy	141 cal
Glycemic Index	low

LENTILS

Lentils may be red, green, or brown. They are a staple food for vegetarians and feature in such classic nonmeat alternatives as baked lentil loaf. They may be added to soups, stews, casseroles, flans, and rissoles. They are used in Asia to make dhal

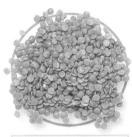

which, if served with rice, provides a balanced intake of amino acids.

Lentils contain useful amounts of important minerals such as copper, iron, zinc, potassium, magnesium, and selenium as well as B vitamins. Red lentils contain small amounts of carotenoid pigments, which are important for their antioxidant properties.

Nutritional values per 100 g RED LENTILS (COOKED)	
Carbohydrate	18 g
Starch	16 g
Sugars	2 g
Protein	8 g
Fat	<1 g
Energy	100 cal
Glycemic Index	low

KIDNEY BEANS

The familiar kidney bean is usually a burgundy red color, but there are also white and black varieties. Kidney beans are a dietary staple in many parts of the world, such as Central America. Soaking this type of bean overnight reduces the cooking time and indigestibility.

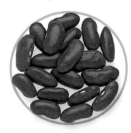

Kidney beans provide twice as much fiber as green beans. In addition, they are a good source of potassium and contain useful amounts of folate,

calcium, magnesium, iron, zinc, and selenium.

Dried kidney beans should always be boiled rapidly for at least 15 minutes, then simmered until thoroughly cooked. This deactivates certain substances (lectins) in them that can otherwise lead to indigestion and symptoms that resemble food poisoning even if very few beans are eaten. Interestingly, lectins have been found to prevent the attachment of disease-causing bacteria, fungi, and viruses to body-cell walls, and these are known as antiadhesins. The lectin that occurs in red kidney beans has been found during research in the laboratory to have a powerful anti-HIV action and is currently under further investigation.

Nutritional values per 100 g KIDNEY BEANS (COOKED)	
Carbohydrate	17 g
Starch	15 g
Sugars	2 g
Protein	8 g
Fat	<1 g
Energy	103 cal
Glycemic Index	low

FRESH FRUIT

Rich carbohydrate source ◆ Provides vitamins, minerals, protective plant nutrients ◆ Good source of fiber

AVOCADO

Avocados are often assumed to be vegetables, but in fact they are fruits. Unlike most fruits, however, an avocado only starts to ripen and fulfill its nutritional potential once it is cut from the tree. Avocados are very versatile, appearing in appetizers or salads. They can also be cooked, for example, in a vegetable and cheese bake.

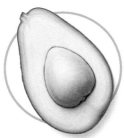

An average-sized avocado weighs about 130 g and provides approximately 250 kcals of energy. A large avocado can supply as much as 400 kcals of

energy. Some varieties provide as much as 80 percent of their energy potential in the form of vegetable oil, mostly monounsaturated fatty acids. These are a rich source of energy and, like those found in olive oil, have beneficial effects on blood cholesterol levels and the circulatory system. Avocados also contain a sugar known as manoheptulose, which helps to satisfy the sensation of hunger.

Nutritional values per 100 g
AVOCADO

Carbohydrate	2 g
Starch	1 g
Sugars	1 g
Protein	2 g
Fat	20 g
Energy	190 kcal
Glycemic Index	low

BANANA

Bananas are the ultimate healthy snack. They can be sliced onto cereal, into lowfat yogurt or custard, or even made into a sandwich filling.

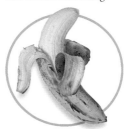

In addition to boosting energy levels generally, bananas have a beneficial effect on mental energy levels. They are a source of the building blocks of the neurotransmitters serotonin and dopamine in the brain. Serotonin is a feel-good substance, while dopamine is important for emotional balance. Bananas are also one of the few foods able to boost sexual energy. They contain bufotenine, which increases your sex drive.

Bananas also contain potassium, magnesium, vitamins B_6, and C.

Nutritional values per 100 g
BANANA

Carbohydrate	23 g
Starch	2 g
Sugars	21 g
Protein	1 g
Fat	<1 g
Energy	95 cal
Glycemic Index	high

GRAPES

Black grapes have long been associated with good health, traditionally being given to patients to speed their recovery. They have energizing fruit sugars and are easy to digest.

Grape sugars are readily fermented to form

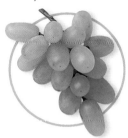

alcohol. Alcohol provides 7 cal of energy per gram, more than protein and carbohydrate but less than fat. Alcohol is readily metabolized but should be drunk in moderation.

National Institutes of Health guidelines about

drinking recommend a limit of two units of alcohol a day for men and one for women. (A unit is defined as half a pint of beer, one ounce of hard liquor, or a small glass of wine.) More than this is inadvisable because of health risks. Women who are pregnant or planning to be should avoid drinking alcohol.

Nutritional values per 100 g GRAPES	
Carbohydrate	15 g
Starch	0 g
Sugars	15 g
Protein	<1 g
Fat	<1 g
Energy	60 cal
Glycemic Index	medium

OLIVES

All olives start off green. As they ripen, their color changes through various shades of purple to black, their flavor mellows, and the percentage of energy-rich oil increases. Olives for making olive oil are picked while they are still unripe. These taste bitter and are totally inedible.

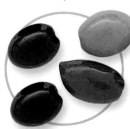

They have a low acid content, which is very important: the lower the acidity, the better the oil.

Olive oil is used for cooking and for drizzling over pizzas, pastas, and

breads, as well as in salad dressings. A diet rich in olive oil has been shown to reduce the risk of coronary artery disease by 25 percent. In a study of more than 600 people recovering from a heart attack, those following a Mediterranean-style diet were found to be 56 percent less likely to suffer another heart attack, or to die from other heart problems, than those eating a normal diet.

In a study of people with high blood pressure, those using 30–40 g of olive oil a day for cooking reduced their need for antihypertensive drugs by almost 50 percent in six months, compared with 4 percent for those using sunflower oil.

Nutritional values per 100 g OLIVES	
Carbohydrate	0 g
Starch	- g
Sugars	- g
Protein	1 g
Fat	11 g
Energy	103 cal
Glycemic Index	low

MANGO

This highly nutritious tropical fruit has a large, flat stone running lengthways down the middle, pungent-tasting skin, and fibrous, slippery flesh that can make it difficult to eat. The best way to prepare it is to slice it lengthways into thirds, discard the central part containing the stone, and to score the flesh of

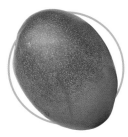

each outer part into a crisscross pattern. If these outer sections are turned inside out, the flesh is presented in bite-sized cubes that are easy to remove. Dried mango slices are increasingly available and provide an energy-filled, delicious, easy-to-eat instant snack.

Mangoes are an excellent source of plant pigments – or carotenoids – some of which the body can convert into vitamin A (retinol). Some

varieties of mango contain as much as 3 g of carotenoid pigment per 100 g of flesh.

Mangoes contain certain substances that are believed to have anti-cancer properties. These are currently the subject of further investigation. Mangoes also contain good amounts of vitamin C and fiber, plus useful amounts of potassium and vitamin E.

Nutritional values per 100 g	
MANGO	
Carbohydrate	14 g
Starch	<1 g
Sugars	14 g
Protein	<1 g
Fat	<1 g
Energy	57 cal
Glycemic Index	medium

PINEAPPLE

When ripe, pineapples consist of about 10 percent fruit sugars and provide a sweet, energy-packed accompaniment to savories such as cheese. They are also an

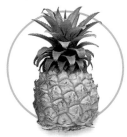

important component of sweet and sour sauces. Unsweetened pineapple juice is a refreshing, energy-boosting drink.

Canker sores are often indicative of a lack of energy and of being generally rundown. The

exact cause of these sores is not known, but a traditional folk remedy is to hold a piece of fresh pineapple flesh against the sore for a while. The bromelain quickly soothes discomfort and promotes healing. Gargling with pineapple juice is a natural remedy that relieves sore throats. In addition, pineapples are a useful source of vitamin C as well as potassium.

Nutritional values per 100 g	
PINEAPPLE	
Carbohydrate	10 g
Starch	0 g
Sugars	10 g
Protein	<1 g
Fat	<1 g
Energy	41 cal
Glycemic Index	low

CHERRIES

A handful of cherries makes a delicious, healthy, and energizing snack, but the small pits can be a choking hazard.

Cherries contain a number of important phytochemicals. These

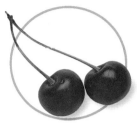

include ellagic acid, which is believed to protect against cancer by blocking the action of an enzyme that may promote the growth of cancer cells.

In addition, cherries are a good source of vitamin C and provide useful amounts of potassium.

Nutritional values per 100 g	
CHERRIES	
Carbohydrate	12 g
Starch	0 g
Sugars	12 g
Protein	1 g
Fat	<1 g
Energy	48 cal
Glycemic Index	low

CITRUS FRUITS

Citrus fruits such as oranges, lemons, limes, and grapefruit are renowned as excellent sources of vitamin C. A single fruit can provide the recommended daily amount of 60 mg a day.

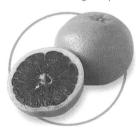

Oranges contain bioflavonoids, powerful antioxidants that help protect against cancer, inflammatory diseases, and heart disease. They also contain the flavonoid hesperidin, while grapefruit contain naringenin. These plant nutrients boost the antioxidant action of vitamin C. Lemons are a rich source of limonoids and limonene – other phytochemicals that may protect against cancer.

Citrus fruits have also been found to help relieve

inflammation, and a good intake of citrus fruits may prevent the irritation of the respiratory airways associated with asthma. Children who eat citrus fruit on most days in winter are less likely to wheeze. The prevention of bronchospasm helps maintain optimum levels of oxygen in the lungs, thereby ensuring that adequate amounts of oxygen are available throughout the body to "burn" fuel such as glucose and fatty acids and provide energy.

Finally, citrus fruits contain pectin, a soluble fiber that helps reduce cholesterol levels, and useful amounts of folate, potassium, and calcium.

Nutritional values per 100 g	
GRAPEFRUIT	
Carbohydrate	7 g
Starch	0 g
Sugars	7 g
Protein	1 g
Fat	<1 g
Energy	30 cal
Glycemic Index	low

DRIED FRUIT

Convenient energy-boosting snack foods ◆ High-fiber

foods ◆ Good source of certain minerals

APRICOTS

Dried apricots are a convenient energy-rich snack. They are highly nutritious and have been included in astronauts' rations. Increasingly

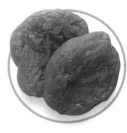

popular are partially dried apricots.

Avoid dried apricots that have been treated with sulfur dioxide (E220) to preserve their rich orange color; this can trigger wheeziness in people with asthma.

A substance in apricot kernels, amygdalin, may be broken down into hydrogen cyanide in the stomach, and cases of fatal poisoning from eating apricot pits have occurred. Extracts of apricot kernels have been used by some alternative practitioners to treat cancer but this is highly controversial.

Nutritional values per 100 g	
READY-TO-EAT APRICOTS	
Carbohydrate	37 g
Starch	0 g
Sugars	37 g
Protein	4 g
Fat	1 g
Energy	158 cal
Glycemic Index	high

FIGS

Fresh, ripe black or green figs are delicious and nutritious, but they bruise easily and do not travel well. Most are therefore sold dried or semidried. Dried figs have about five or six times the energy value of fresh figs because the water has been removed and the sugar

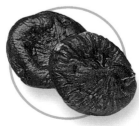

KEY BENEFITS
Dried or semidried figs are an excellent snack for raising blood sugar levels quickly and are convenient to carry around for a quick energy boost. They consist of more than 50 percent sugar by weight, most of which is glucose and fructose.

content concentrated. The sugar content is so high, it is best to brush your teeth after eating figs.

Figs consist of 8 percent fiber and have a gentle laxative action enhanced by a substance known as mucin. Dried figs are a rich source of potassium and calcium (gram for gram, even more than milk), as well as iron and magnesium.

The fig has long had a reputation for boosting sexual energy levels. The fruit is considered to be highly erotic and the juicy, pale pink flesh of a cut fig is said to resemble the female genitalia.

Nutritional values per 100 g	
DRIED FIGS	
Carbohydrate	53 g
Starch	0 g
Sugars	53 g
Protein	4 g
Fat	2 g
Energy	227 cal
Glycemic Index	high

DATES

Dates are the fruit of a tropical palm. They vary from shiny brown to honey colored, while some are distinctly red. Traditionally, dried dates were a staple convenience food of the nomadic

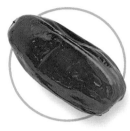

cultures of North Africa and the Near East. They can be eaten for several months after harvesting and sun-drying. Up to 110 lbs (50 kg) can be harvested from a mature date palm. They are an easily transportable source of carbohydrate, and are often called "the bread of the desert."

Dates are a good source of potassium and contain useful amounts of calcium, magnesium, iron, selenium, and the

B-group vitamins. Dried dates contain virtually no vitamin C and should ideally be eaten with a vitamin-C source such as orange juice in order to enhance the absorption of their iron.

Dates combine well with other fruit, cheese, and nuts. Chilling them for an hour first makes slicing them much easier.

• CAUTION

Dates contain tyramine which may trigger a migraine in some people.

Nutritional values per 100 g	
DATES	
Carbohydrate	57 g
Starch	0 g
Sugars	57 g
Protein	3 g
Fat	<1 g
Energy	227 cal
Glycemic Index	high

PRUNES

Prunes are produced by drying several different varieties of plum, the most popular of which is the d'Agen sugar plum. On average, it takes 8 lbs (3.5 kg) of plums to make 2 lbs (1 kg) of prunes.

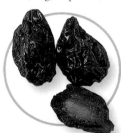

Prunes are a good source of fiber (13 percent) and, ounce for ounce, provide more than dried beans. They are a popular choice at breakfast to maintain

regular bowel action. The laxative action is probably caused by a substance that stimulates the secretion of fluid into the bowels and also encourages intestinal contraction. Prunes may cause gas initially, but if eaten regularly this effect will be reduced as bacteria in the bowel adapt to producing more enzymes needed for digesting fiber.

Prunes are a good source of potassium and contain useful amounts of calcium, magnesium, iron, selenium, and B-group vitamins. Prunes are best eaten with a vitamin-C source in order to maximize absorption of the iron.

Prunes also have a reputation for boosting sexual energy and they used to be served to both workers and clients in medieval brothels.

Nutritional values per 100 g	
PRUNES	
Carbohydrate	34 g
Starch	0 g
Sugars	34 g
Protein	3 g
Fat	<1 g
Energy	141 cal
Glycemic Index	high

OILY FISH

Excellent source of essential fats ◆ Supply many vitamins
and minerals ◆ Protect against heart disease

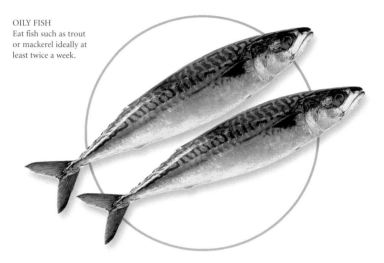

OILY FISH
Eat fish such as trout
or mackerel ideally at
least twice a week.

ESSENTIAL OILS

Oily fishes such as salmon, mackerel, trout, sardines, and herrings are a rich source of omega-3 essential fatty acids, which provide an ideal fuel for powering muscle cells.

A lack of essential fatty acids has been linked to a lack of energy. In studies, as many as 80 percent of those people suffering from chronic fatigue benefitted from high doses of omega-3 fish oils. Interestingly, research has indicated that fish oils may reduce insulin secretion in those with diabetes (types I and II), thus increasing blood sugar levels. If you have diabetes and wish to take fish-oil supplements, monitor your blood sugar levels regularly in case your medication needs to be changed.

OIL CHANGE

If you do not like eating fish, you can take capsules containing omega-3 fish oils instead. Emulsified oils help prevent the fishy aftertaste that some people find distasteful. Staple foods such as margarine, bread, and even milk fortified with refined fish oil are now available to help boost intakes of those people who do not eat much fish. Natural fish oils contain little vitamin E and can go rancid easily. When buying fish-oil capsules, choose those preparations fortified with vitamin E.

KEY BENEFITS

Fish oils are a very rich source of two derivatives of an essential fatty acid (alpha-linolenic), eicosapentanoic acid and docosahexaenoic acid (EPA and DHA for short). They have a thinning effect on the blood (reducing the risk of blood clots), reduce cholesterol, and prevent coronary artery disease (CAD). Eating oily fish two or three times a week may reduce the risk of developing CAD more significantly than by following a lowfat, high-fiber diet.

NUTS & SEEDS

Good source of unsaturated fats, protein, and minerals

◆ Many health-giving properties

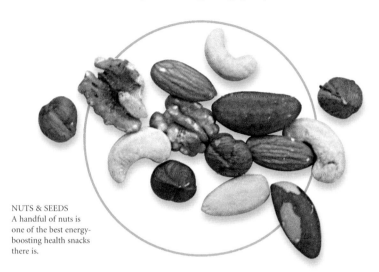

NUTS & SEEDS
A handful of nuts is
one of the best energy-
boosting health snacks
there is.

VITAL NUTRIENTS

Nuts and seeds are a rich source of energy in the form of fatty acids. Many are processed to obtain nutritionally valuable oils.

Almost all nuts and seeds are good sources of estrogen-like plant nutrients. Linseed is the richest known dietary source of phytoestrogens, called lignans. Eating 1 oz (25 g) of linseed a day may shrink estrogen-sensitive tumors pre-operatively. Eating nuts and seeds is especially beneficial at menopause.

PREVENTING DISEASE

Just 2 oz (50 g) of walnuts a day may help reduce blood cholesterol and protect against heart disease. Walnuts also contain antioxidants such as selenium and vitamin E. Brazil nuts are the richest source of selenium with 5,300 mcg per 100 g.

Fresh peanuts are a good source of another antioxidant, resveratrol, believed to protect against coronary heart disease.

Nuts also provide fiber: there are 6 g of fiber in 4 oz (100 g) of walnuts. Also, sesame seeds and peanuts are believed to boost sexual energy levels.

• CAUTION
Some people are highly allergic to nut protein.

SEED & NUT MIX

4 oz (100 g) mixed unsalted nuts
2 oz (50 g) each of sunflower seeds (toasted and/or raw), pumpkin seeds (toasted and/or raw), pine nuts, sesame seeds (toasted), and poppy seeds

Mix all the ingredients well and sprinkle onto salads or rice dishes as desired.

KEY BENEFITS

Fatty acids form the basis of energy production in muscle cells. Those in nuts include the important omega-3 fatty acids. Eat 1 oz (30 g) of nuts or seeds daily for hormone balance, healthy skin, circulation, immunity, and for moderating inflammatory reactions.

FOOD FOR
ALL-DAY ENERGY

Your energy levels will dip at some part of the day, especially if you lead a very busy life. Make sure you grab something healthy and truly energy-giving when you feel hungry, and prepare high-energy dishes at mealtimes.

1 Drink at least 70–100 fl. oz (2–3 liters) of fluid a day. This can be tap or bottled water, mineral water, tea, or unsweetened fruit juice. Carry a small bottle of water around with you at all times and drink from it frequently. By the time you feel thirsty you are already dehydrated and dehydration saps energy. Green tea is a particularly energizing drink since it contains catechins, substances that speed up the body's metabolic rate so that more energy is produced.

2 For an instantly energizing snack, eat a handful of mixed dried fruit (such as apricots, figs, dates, and raisins), nuts, and seeds. Make up a jar containing your favorite mix and keep it within reach. This is a much healthier option than opening the cookie jar.

4 Eat pasta at least once or twice a week. Remember that whole-wheat varieties provide extra fiber, vitamins, and minerals. Avoid serving pasta in a rich sauce. Choose a simple accompaniment such as tomato and basil sauce or a spoonful of red or green pesto.

3 Rather than buying a pastry on your way to work for a midmorning snack, take a bag of fresh fruit with you. A banana, for example, will keep you going well. Whenever you feel hungry, grab an apple or a handful of dried fruit such as ready-to-eat apricots.

5 Always eat breakfast. Sugar-free breakfast cereals, granola, oatmeal, or whole-wheat toast plus yogurt, fresh fruit, and unsweetened fruit juice give you a great start to the day. Yeast extract, a rich source of energizing B-group vitamins, makes a delicious, distinctive-tasting spread on toast.

6

A high-energy salad, served with a whole-grain roll, makes a healthy lunch and a great change from a sandwich. Possible mixtures include cold whole-wheat pasta and corn; egg, mustard, and watercress; mixed bean; green, yellow, and red pepper; or mesclun with fennel and celery.

7

Try to eat vegetarian meals several times a week. These are energizing and are also packed with vitamins, minerals, and protective plant nutrients. Select appetizing recipes such as spinach and mushroom lasagna, Mediterranean tomato and bean casserole, or cheese and lentil loaf. There are thousands of vegetarian recipes these days and many of them are quick and easy to prepare.

8

Oily fish are an important source of essential fatty acids as well as protein, which together make fish an excellent energy source. Cook fish by broiling, steaming, baking in foil or paper, or by poaching. Lightly brush with olive oil if necessary, and serve with freshly squeezed lemon juice and a few freshly chopped herbs.

9

Invest in a juicer and prepare your own delicious fresh fruit and vegetable juices packed with vitamins, minerals, antioxidants, and energizing, natural fruit sugars. Freshly prepared juices have a creamy texture, a milky hue, and provide a wonderful taste experience. They are an exceptionally rich source of nutrients as a result of their concentration: $3\frac{1}{2}$ fluid oz (100 ml) of carrot juice, for example, provides as many carotenoids as 8 oz (225 g) of raw carrots. Try different mixes such as orange and strawberry; melon and raspberry; grape, apricot, passionfruit, and mango; carrot and tangerine; cucumber, beet, and tomato; or avocado, carrot, and orange.

10

Serve oat crackers or rice cakes in place of sweet or salty crackers or cookies with cheese and fruit at the end of a meal or for a snack. Oats and rice are among the best energy-boosting foods.

GETTING NUTRITIONAL HELP

How can you be sure that your diet is providing all the
essential nutrients that your body needs? How best can
you replenish low stocks and thus boost energy levels?
Who can answer these questions for you?

WHO DOES WHAT

Advice about what to eat may be
obtained from a dietician or
nutritionist and information about
nutritional supplements is available
from a nutritional therapist. See
page 70 for general guidelines about
taking supplements. Never take
so-called mega-doses or exceed the
manufacturer's recommended
dosage without taking advice. Either
course of action may be harmful.

DIETICIANS AND NUTRITIONISTS

If you have a diet-related health
problem, such as obesity, diabetes
or a high level of blood cholesterol,
your doctor may refer you to a
dietician or nutritionist for advice
about your particular problem.
Alternatively, you may find one
yourself through the referral service
of the American Dietetic Association. Dieticians are licensed in 41
states, although the regulations vary.
All registered dieticians (RD) have
to complete accreditation require-
ments and any ongoing professional
development for the state(s) in
which they are licensed to practice.

NATUROPATHIC PHYSICIANS

As an alternative to a physician, you
may choose to consult a doctor of
naturopathic medicine (ND). These
primary health care practitioners,
who have graduated from a four-
year accredited naturopathic
program, provide general health
care and advice on staying healthy.
Like medical doctors, they can
diagnose and treat acute and
chronic conditions. Naturopaths are
trained in all modern diagnostic
methods, but, wherever possible,
they avoid the use of most synthetic
drugs as well as major surgery. They
may specialize in one or more areas,
such as nutrition; herbal, physical,
or oriental medicine (including
acupuncture); homeopathy; or
naturopathic obstetrics.

PHARMACISTS

If you are taking prescribed or over-
the-counter medications and are
not sure whether they may interact
with each other or with an herbal
preparation, a pharmacist should be
able to advise you about possible
adverse effects, or refer you to your
doctor if necessary.

ENERGY SUPPLEMENTS

DIETARY SOURCES OF IMPORTANT NUTRIENTS SHOULD ALWAYS BE YOUR FIRST CHOICE, BUT THERE ARE TIMES WHEN A VITAMIN AND MINERAL SUPPLEMENT CAN ACT AS A USEFUL NUTRITIONAL SAFETY NET. IN ADDITION, MANY HERBAL SUPPLEMENTS HAVE THE POTENTIAL TO BOOST YOUR PHYSICAL, MENTAL AND SEXUAL ENERGY LEVELS IF YOU FEEL THEY ARE NOT AS HIGH AS THEY SHOULD BE.

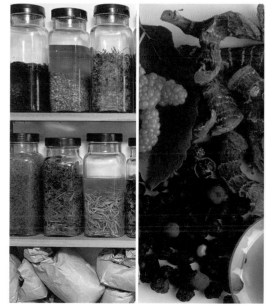

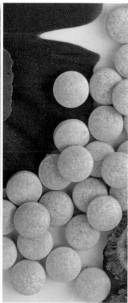

TAKING SUPPLEMENTS

Supplements that boost your metabolism and improve the way your body systems work can increase your energy levels and help you attain optimum health. Energy-boosting supplements work in a variety of different ways.

THE IMPORTANCE OF ENERGY-BOOSTING SUPPLEMENTS

- They have a direct stimulatory effect on the central nervous system, increasing alertness and concentration; for example, guarana
- They improve blood circulation to the brain, increasing the supply of oxygen and nutrients; for example, ginkgo
- They boost the production of energy inside body cells; for example, the B-group vitamins and magnesium
- They stimulate adrenal function; for example, vitamin B_5, magnesium, and ginseng
- They improve immunity by increasing white cell function and resistance to infection; for example, ginseng and propolis

---

NUTRIENT DEFICIENCES

One of the most common causes of a lack of energy is a mild deficiency in the vitamins and minerals needed for energy-producing metabolic reactions. Deficiency may be due to poor diet, a reduced ability to absorb micronutrients from the gut, or the fact that nutrients are being used up more quickly than usual so the amount needed is greater. Increased usage happens if the body is under stress, for example, when B-group vitamins and antioxidants such as vitamin C are rapidly depleted.

Many people who are fatigued look for a quick energy boost such as that provided by a cup of coffee. However, too much caffeine may ultimately cause a lack of energy as well as other symptoms such as restlessness, insomnia, headaches, and anxiety. It is much better in fact to use a gentler energy-boosting substance such as guarana, which contains a substance very similar to caffeine, or a supplement that acts as an adaptogen.

Vitamin C is vitally important in food, such as vegetables and fruit, or as a daily supplement.

ADAPTOGENS

An adaptogen is a substance that strengthens, normalizes and regulates body systems. It has wide-ranging benefits and boosts energy levels as a consequence.

Adaptogens increase the production of energy in body cells by making the uptake of oxygen and the processing of cell wastes more efficient. This encourages cell growth and increases cell survival. Adaptogens have been shown to normalize blood-sugar levels and hormone synthesis, and to counter the detrimental effects of stress and disrupted biorhythms.

Adaptogens seem to work best as an energy stimulant if fatigue results not from physical exertion but from an underlying problem such as poor diet, hormone imbalance, stress, or excesses of caffeine, nicotine, or alcohol. Lifestyle changes may also be required therefore to maximize their benefits. If taken with vitamins C and B-complex, the effects of adaptogens may also be improved.

THREE-STEP SUPPLEMENT PROGRAM

1 Take a good multivitamin and mineral supplement to safeguard against nutrient deficiencies. Choose one containing as many vitamins and minerals as possible and providing 100 percent of the RDI (Reference Daily Intake).

Multivitamin and mineral supplement

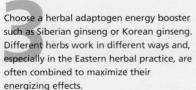

2 Take evening primrose oil or fish oil capsules to provide essential fatty acids, which are vital for good health and energy production. In trials, essential fatty acids have been shown to a have significant beneficial effect on 70–80 percent of people suffering from chronic fatigue.

Evening primrose and herb capsules

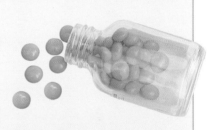

3 Choose a herbal adaptogen energy booster such as Siberian ginseng or Korean ginseng. Different herbs work in different ways and, especially in the Eastern herbal practice, are often combined to maximize their energizing effects.

Herbal adaptogen in capsule form

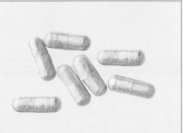

VITAMIN SUPPLEMENTS

Boost energy-generating metabolic processes ◆ Prevent vitamin deficiencies ◆ Protect against disease

VITAMIN C
RDI: **60 MG**

Vitamin C is a powerful antioxidant that suppresses energy-draining inflammation

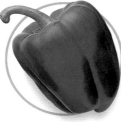

in the body. It acts as an essential cofactor in at least 300 metabolic reactions, including many involved in energy production. It is essential for the synthesis of collagen – a major structural protein – and for the growth, repair, and reproduction of healthy tissue. Vitamin C also increases the absorption of iron, which is needed to make the oxygen-carrying red blood pigment, hemoglobin. An iron supplement washed down with orange juice will ensure that more iron is absorbed and less passes out of the body unused.

Vitamin C also has antiviral properties and is used to treat or help prevent the common cold and the flu. Studies show that it can reduce the severity of symptoms and the duration of a cold by 20 percent and – for some people – lessen the risk of infection after exposure to a cold virus. Adaptogens such as ginseng seem to work better if vitamin C is being taken as well, but the two should ideally be taken hours apart.

SYMPTOMS OF DEFICIENCY
- ◆ Lack of energy
- ◆ Frequent colds and other infections
- ◆ Weakness
- ◆ Muscle and joint pain
- ◆ Wounds heal slowly
- ◆ Bleeding gums

VITAMIN E
RDI: **20 MG**

Vitamin E is another powerful antioxidant that protects against harmful effects of free radicals. It protects cell membranes, nerve sheaths, circulating cholesterol molecules, dietary fats, and body fat stores from damage by oxidation and rancidity.

This vitamin also has a strengthening effect on muscle fibers, relieving muscle cramps, and improves skin healing and suppleness. Vitamin E also boosts immunity (by working with selenium to increase the production of antibodies) and seems to

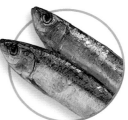

improve the body's use of glucose, thus improving energy production.

If you are taking a vitamin E supplement, select one described as a natural source (d-alpha tocopherol) which will have greater bioactivity. Amounts of vitamin E are sometimes expressed in international units rather than milligrams: 1.5 IU is the equivalent of 1 mg.

SYMPTOMS OF DEFICIENCY
- ◆ Lethargy
- ◆ Poor concentration
- ◆ Irritability
- ◆ Reduced sex drive
- ◆ Muscle weakness
- ◆ Poor coordination

B-GROUP VITAMINS

The B-group vitamins play an important role in more than 60 different metabolic reactions involving the processing of carbohydrates, fats, and protein. They are particularly involved in energy production itself and the synthesis of glucose and fatty acids, both of which are very

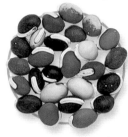

important "fuels" for the powering of muscle cells.

B-group vitamins are also crucially involved in the transmission of messages between nerve cells and muscle cells, and are very important for the manufacture of red blood cells, which carry oxygen around in the bloodstream. Good circulation of oxygen around the body is absolutely essential for the efficient production of energy in muscles.

RDIs

Vitamin B_1 (thiamine)	1.5 mg
Vitamin B_2 (riboflavin)	1.7 mg
Vitamin B_3 (niacin)	20 mg
Vitamin B_5 (pantothenic acid)	10 mg
Vitamin B_6 (pyridoxine)	2 mg
Vitamin B_{12} (cyanocobalamin)	6 mcg
Biotin	0.3 mg
Folic acid	400 mcg

FEEL-GOOD VITAMIN

Vitamin B_1, or thiamine, has a beneficial effect on mood, helping you feel more calm, agreeable, clear-headed, elated, and energetic. People with low levels of thiamine are less likely to feel self-confident and more likely to suffer from depression than those with adequate levels of thiamine. Many people, in fact, do have low intakes of thiamine. Eating whole-grain cereal for breakfast, or taking B_1 supplements, can help increase your feelings of general well-being and relieve fatigue, especially in older people. In one trial, those taking 10 mg of vitamin B_1 daily enjoyed better-quality sleep, more energy, and lower blood pressure than those who took a placebo.

CONVERTING ENERGY

Vitamins B_2 and B_5 are needed for converting the calories obtained from carbohydrates, fats, and protein into a form of energy that can be used by body cells. B_3 enables energy to be released from digested food. B_6 is concerned particularly with the metabolism of protein.

MAKING NEW CELLS

B_{12} is involved in the production of healthy red blood cells and also in controlling the appetite. Together with another B-group vitamin, folate, it is needed for making new genetic material (DNA) during cell division. The vitamin is most needed by cells with a rapid turnover such as those lining the gut (which are shed about every three days), cells in hair follicles, and bone marrow, which produces new red blood cells. A lack of vitamin B_{12} or folate causes the production of cells that are larger than they should be. In the case of red blood cells, this leads to a particular form of anemia known as pernicious anemia. This condition develops slowly and symptoms are often not recognized until an advanced stage, but common indications are fatigue and lack of energy.

People with chronic fatigue syndrome often benefit from taking vitamin B supplements. Preliminary research suggests their level of B vitamin activity is low.

SYMPTOMS OF DEFICIENCY

- Fatigue
- Paleness (anemia)
- Headaches
- Loss of appetite
- Irritability
- Loss of concentration
- Poor memory
- Difficulty sleeping
- Difficulty coping with stress
- Depression
- Muscle weakness and stiffness
- Nerve tingling, burning, and numbness

MINERAL SUPPLEMENTS

Prevent mineral deficiencies ◆ Boost energy-producing metabolic processes ◆ Protect against disease

CHROMIUM

There is no RDI set for chromium but intakes of 50–200 mcg a day are generally considered both safe and adequate.

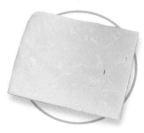

Only one chemical form of chromium can be used in the body. Minute amounts are needed to form an organic complex known as the Glucose Tolerance Factor (GTF). This substance interacts with the hormone insulin to regulate the uptake of glucose by cells and thus encourage the production of energy from glucose, especially in muscle cells.

Little chromium is to be found in most refined carbohydrates. Also, if your diet is high in sugar, you are more likely to lose chromium in your urine. Chromium deficiency is thought to affect as many as 90 percent of the adult population. The foods that should be included in the diet in order to replenish stocks of this mineral (and help with weight control) are egg yolks, red meat, cheese, whole grains, yeast, legumes, and nuts.

> ### SYMPTOMS OF DEFICIENCY
> ◆ Lack of energy
> ◆ Muscle weakness
> ◆ Poor glucose tolerance and diabetes
> ◆ Poor tolerance of alcohol
> ◆ Hunger pangs and weight gain
> ◆ Irritability and depression
> ◆ Excessive thirst
> ◆ Dizziness

IODINE
RDI: 150 MCG

This mineral is needed by the thyroid gland for the production of two thyroid hormones, thyroxine and

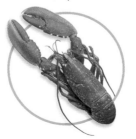

tri-iodothyronine. Both hormones are involved in regulating the speed of the body's metabolism, and hence the rate at which energy food is digested and energy is subsequently generated.

If your diet does not include many dairy foods or seafood, you may be lacking iodine. Good food sources include marine fish, for example tuna, haddock, and halibut; seafood, such as shrimp, mussels, lobsters, and oysters; seaweed such as kelp; iodized salt; milk (cattle feed is iodized); and crops grown and meat obtained from livestock reared on soils exposed to sea spray.

> ### SYMPTOMS OF DEFICIENCY
> ◆ Underactive thyroid gland
> ◆ Swollen thyroid gland (goiter)
> ◆ Fatigue
> ◆ Lack of energy
> ◆ Muscle weakness
> ◆ Susceptibility to the cold
> ◆ Weight gain
> ◆ Coarse skin and brittle hair
> ◆ Poor concentration

IRON
RDI: **10** MG

Iron is essential for the manufacture of the red blood pigment, hemoglobin, which

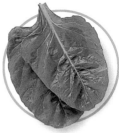

transports oxygen around the body. Iron also occurs in a protein, myoglobin, which binds oxygen in muscle cells and helps maintain muscle stamina. In addition, this mineral is a cofactor in many metabolic reactions involving the generation of energy and the proper functioning of the body's immune system.

You can maintain iron supplies by including the following foods in your diet: shellfish, brewer's yeast, organ meats, red meat, fish (especially sardines), egg yolk, green vegetables, wheat germ, whole-wheat bread, and dried fruit.

SYMPTOMS OF
DEFICIENCY
♦ Paleness (anemia)
♦ Fatigue
♦ Muscle fatigue
♦ Dizziness
♦ Sore tongue and cracking at the corners of the mouth
♦ Fast pulse
♦ Shortness of breath

MAGNESIUM
RDI: **400** MG

Magnesium is found in all body tissues and maintains the electrical stability of cells. This includes the regulation of the heartbeat. Magnesium is important for every major metabolic reaction in the body, from the synthesis of proteins and genetic material to the production of energy from glucose. It is also

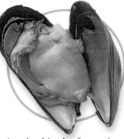

involved in the formation and reactions of more than 300 enzymes, so it is important for most body systems to function well.

Good food sources of magnesium to be included in the diet are seafood, seaweed, meat, eggs, dairy products, whole grains, bananas, apricots, dark green leafy vegetables, soybeans, nuts and seeds, and brewer's yeast.

SYMPTOMS OF
DEFICIENCY
♦ Weakness
♦ Fatigue
♦ Loss of appetite
♦ Muscle trembling and cramps
♦ Loss of coordination
♦ Premenstrual syndrome
♦ Nausea

PHOSPHORUS
RDI: **1** G

Phosphorus is involved in the production of energy-storage molecules (ATP and ADP, *see page 11*) in muscle cells, and is needed to activate B-group vitamins in the generation

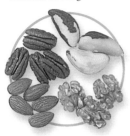

of energy. Phosphate is therefore important for optimizing athletic performance. Taking supplements for three days before a competition can increase the time to exhaustion by 20 percent. Other studies suggest that phosphate supplements can increase maximal power output by as much as 17 percent.

Phosphorus is found in many foods so symptoms of deficiency do not commonly occur.

SYMPTOMS OF
DEFICIENCY
♦ General malaise
♦ Lack of energy
♦ Loss of appetite
♦ Increased susceptibility to infection
♦ Anemia
♦ Muscle weakness
♦ Numbness or pins and needles
♦ Irritability
♦ Confusion

POTASSIUM

There is no RDI set for potassium but an intake of about 2,000 mg daily is advisable. It is estimated, however, that one in three people receive less potassium than this. Potassium is the main

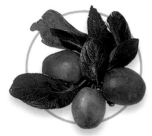

positively charged ion inside cells, where it is present in concentrations 30 times greater than in the extracellular fluid surrounding cells. This difference between cells and their surroundings is responsible for the body's bioelectromagnetic field. This is essential for muscle contraction, nerve conduction, maintaining blood sugar levels and the production of proteins.

Potassium is found in a variety of fresh and dried fruit and vegetables, seafood and whole grains.

SYMPTOMS OF DEFICIENCY
♦ Lack of energy
♦ Poor appetite
♦ Fatigue
♦ Weakness
♦ Muscle cramps
♦ Irregular heartbeat
♦ Irritability
♦ Pins and needles
♦ Drowsiness and confusion

SELENIUM

There is no RDI but an intake of 60 mg daily is essential for cell growth and for the immune system to function. It is important for healthy muscle fibers – including those of the heart – and is also needed to regulate the production of a thyroid hormone, tri-iodothyronine. If iodine

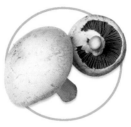

and selenium intakes are both low, there is a greater risk of an underactive thyroid and, subsequently, low energy levels.

Most people get an adequate amount in their diet. Selenium is found in many vegetables, such as asparagus, broccoli, celery, mushrooms, garlic, cabbage, radishes, and onions. It also occurs in nuts, whole grains, eggs, and seafood, as well as brewer's yeast.

SYMPTOMS OF DEFICIENCY
♦ Muscle weakness
♦ Lack of energy (if thyroid function is reduced)
♦ Frequent infections
♦ Low male fertility
♦ Poor prostate health
♦ Signs of premature aging

ZINC
RDI: 15 MG

Zinc is essential for the action of more than 100 enzymes involved in the functioning of most of the body's systems. This mineral is particularly important for growth, sexual maturity, wound

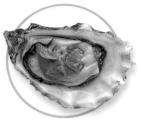

healing, immunity, the detoxification of harmful substances, and the release of insulin.

If your diet includes an adequate amount of protein you will be getting plenty of zinc. Good dietary sources of zinc include red meat, seafood (especially oysters), organ meats (liver in particular), whole grains, brewer's yeast, eggs, legumes, and cheese.

SYMPTOMS OF DEFICIENCY
♦ Poor growth
♦ Reduced fertility
♦ Impaired immunity and susceptibility to infection
♦ Loss of taste and sense of smell
♦ Poor appetite
♦ Reduced mental energy levels and slower thinking
♦ Low spirits
♦ Sleep disturbance

NUTRITIONAL SUPPLEMENTS

Boost energy-producing metabolic processes ◆ Protect against disease ◆ Balance hormones

COENZYME Q10

A compound similar to a vitamin, coenzyme Q10 (or CoQ10 as it is known) is essential for cells to process oxygen and to generate energy-rich molecules. It enables energy in food molecules to be converted into a

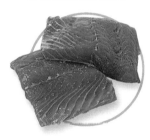

form usable by muscle cells. It improves stamina and endurance, making it popular among athletes, strengthens muscles, and has antioxidant properties.

The optimal dietary intake of CoQ10 is not known. Average adult daily intakes are estimated at 3–5 mg for meateaters and 1 mg for vegetarians.

GOOD FOOD SOURCES

◆ Meat
◆ Fish
◆ Whole grains
◆ Nuts
◆ Green vegetables

Supplements tend to provide 10–100 mg daily, often taken in two doses. CoQ10 is best taken with food, which improves its absorption. Ensure that you also have good intakes of vitamins B and C for the best results.

PROBIOTICS

These "friendly" bacteria, such as *Lactobacilli* and bifidobacteria, are used to promote a good digestive balance. The intestines contain about 11 trillion bacteria. At least 70 percent should be healthy, probiotic types and only 30 percent of the less beneficial variety, but in reality it is often the other way around, so make sure

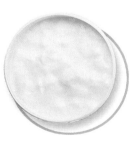

that you take probiotics in dietary or supplementary form every day.

Probiotic bacteria produce lactic acid and are found naturally in the large bowel. They help create a healthy intestinal environment and prevent infection by bacteria, viruses, and yeasts. They compete with harmful bacteria for nutrients and attachment sites on intestinal cell walls. They have also been shown to secrete natural antibiotics and stimulate production of interferon, the body's own antiviral substance. Improved digestion and resistance to infection are important for optimum energy levels.

In addition, *Lactobacilli* are needed by women for the health of the lower reproductive tract, where they protect against recurrent infections that have a draining effect on sexual energy levels.

The use of probiotics includes substances such as fructo-oligosaccharides (FOS) and oatmeal. Dietary sources of natural FOS include barley, wheat, garlic, onions, bananas, honey, and tomatoes.

GOOD FOOD SOURCES

◆ Live yogurt
◆ Fermented milk drinks

ISOFLAVONES

Intakes of at least 2.5 mg to 50 mg of isoflavones daily are recommended.

Isoflavones are a type of plant hormone that have a structure similar to that of human estrogens. The isoflavones that have been most extensively studied (such as genistein, daidzein, formononetin, biochanin A, and glycitein) are found in

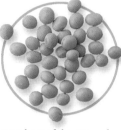

members of the pea and bean family. Typically, 60 g of soy protein yield 45 mg of isoflavones.

Paradoxically, these plant hormones are able to improve both low- and high-estrogen ailments. Isoflavones are about 500 to 1,000 times weaker than human estrogens and can reduce high estrogen levels in the body by competing with stronger estrogens for receptors (attachment sites) in estrogen-sensitive tissues such as the breasts. This therefore reduces the amount of estrogen stimulation a cell receives. Alternatively, isoflavones can provide a useful hormone boost when estrogen levels in the body are low, for example, during and after menopause. Hormone

imbalances are a common cause of depleted physical, mental, and sexual energy.

In parts of the world where dietary intakes of isoflavones are high, such as Japan, there is no word or phrase that means menopausal hot flash, because so few women experience these energy-draining symptoms. In studies of Western women, taking isoflavone supplements has been shown to reduce the number of hot flashes experienced a day by 45 percent over a period of three months, compared with only 30 percent in women taking a placebo.

By correcting both high and low estrogen states, isoflavones help maintain optimum physical, emotional, and sexual energy levels at all stages of adult life. Also beneficial for men, they help maintain a healthy prostate gland and blood circulation.

GOOD FOOD SOURCES
◆ Soybeans
◆ Tofu
◆ Soymilk
◆ Whole grains
◆ Chickpeas

FISH OILS

Typically, intakes of 1–2 g daily are recommended.

Essential fatty acids, or EFAs, are found in fish and plant oils. Some occur in oily fish and others in nuts and seeds (and their oils). Omega-3

fish oils are a rich source of essential fatty acids. These are known to originate in microalgae and become concentrated in fish that feed off large amounts of plankton.

The action of omega-3 polyunsaturated fatty acids balances that of

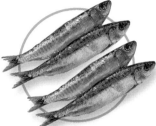

omega-6-polyunsaturated fatty acids, derived mostly from vegetable oils. Omega-3 oils have a protective action against long-term inflammatory diseases such as asthma, rheumatoid arthritis, and psoriasis. Inflammatory conditions are associated with a profound lack of energy, so a fish-oil supplement will help reduce the risk of energy levels falling. As many as 80 percent of people with chronic fatigue have benefitted from taking high doses of omega-3 fish oils together with evening primrose oil, which is rich in omega-6 essential fatty acids.

Interestingly, energy-draining and painful menstrual periods seem to be significantly worse in women who do not eat much fish. Taking omega-3 fish-oil supplements has been shown to relieve painful periods in teenage girls. This is because omega-3 essential fatty acids have a beneficial effect on prostaglandins produced in the womb lining (endometrium), reducing muscle spasm.

Essential fatty acids are also important during pregnancy, helping to improve the development of a baby's eyes and brain. If an expectant mother's diet is lacking in EFAs, her baby will obtain those it needs from her body's richest store – the brain. This may account for the slight shrinkage (2–3 percent) in maternal brain size seen in some pregnant women and the consequential reduced mental energy levels. This results in the lack of concentration, poor memory, forgetfulness, and vagueness that many women experience, especially during the last few months of pregnancy.

If you want to take a fish oil supplement during pregnancy, make sure it is one intended for pregnant women. Avoid cod liver oil supplements that contain vitamin A, excessive amounts of which may be harmful to a developing baby.

GOOD FOOD SOURCES
- ◆ Trout
- ◆ Salmon
- ◆ Herring
- ◆ Mackerel
- ◆ Sardines
- ◆ Anchovies
- ◆ Tuna

ANTIOXIDANTS

Daily intakes of 6 mg of carotenoids, up to 3 g of vitamin C, 30 IU of vitamin E, and 200 mcg of selenium are advisable.

An antioxidant is a protective substance that helps neutralize the damaging effects of chemicals known as free radicals. These are byproducts of the body's metabolic processes in which cells use oxygen to produce energy. A free radical is an unstable molecular fragment that is missing an electron (one of the fundamental

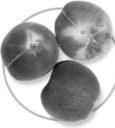

particles making up an atom). Free radicals take electrons from other places, such as body cells, to become stable but damage the other cells in the process. This is an oxidation process. It can trigger chain reactions in which electrons are moved from one molecule to another, damaging fats, proteins, cell membranes, and genetic material. A body cell may undergo as many as 10,000 free-radical oxidations a day. These have been linked to a number of degenerative health problems, many of which have low levels of energy as a symptom.

Antioxidants are the main defense against free-radical attack. They give up one of their own electrons to a free radical, preventing the chain reactions and cell damage.

Several vitamins and minerals are antioxidants. Of these, the most important are vitamin A and beta-carotene (a plant pigment converted by the body into vitamin A), vitamins C and E, and the mineral selenium. Vitamins C and E and selenium are available as one supplement. Other substances that have a lesser antioxidant action but are still important include vitamin B_2, zinc, copper, and manganese.

Other antioxidants are available in supplement form, for example pine bark extracts, coenzyme Q10, bilberry, grapeseed extracts, ginkgo, green tea, and carotenoids such as lutein and lycopene.

GOOD FOOD SOURCES
- ◆ Vitamin A: oily fish, dairy produce, liver
- ◆ Beta-carotene: red peppers, carrots, apricots, dark green leafy vegetables
- ◆ Vitamin C: papaya, blackcurrants, green peppers, broccoli, citrus fruits
- ◆ Vitamin E: wheat-germ oil, sunflower seeds/ oil, nuts, avocado
- ◆ Selenium: nuts, tuna, sunflower seeds, shrimps

ENERGY HERBS

Protect against the debilitating effects of stress ◆ Boost energy levels ◆ Improve general well-being

ASHWAGANDHA

Ashwagandha – known as winter cherry or Indian ginseng – is a restorative tonic in Ayurvedic medicine, boosting energy

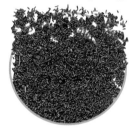

and improving resistance to stress. It is a powerful adaptogen that some people consider superior to Korean ginseng for improve mental acuity and physical performance.

Ashwagandha reduces anxiety and promotes serenity and deep sleep, thus relieving nervous exhaustion and boosting energy. It strengthens muscles and tendons, boosts immunity, and improves concentration.
- CAUTION
See General Guidelines on page 70. Ashwagandha may be difficult to digest.

DOSAGE
Take 150–300 mg daily. Capsules standardized to contain 2–5 mg of withanolides, an important constituent.

BLUE-GREEN ALGAE

Blue-green algae, such as chlorella and spirulina, are a rich source of more than 100 nutrients, such as vitamins, minerals, antioxidants, enzymes, essential fatty acids, and amino acids. Chlorella also contains a unique substance that acts as an energy concentrate.

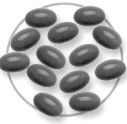

Blue-green algae detoxify by neutralizing toxins. The most potent, purest algae thrive in freshwater free from pollution.
- CAUTION
Use mainstream brands to avoid the risk of contamination from polluted water. See page 70 for General Guidelines.

DOSAGE
Typically, 3 g daily, preferably with food.

GINSENG

Ginseng – usually referred to as Chinese, Korean, or Asian ginseng – is one of

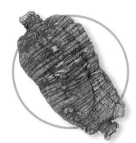

the oldest-known herbal medicines, having been used as a revitalizing, energizing tonic in the East for over 7,000 years.

An adaptogen, ginseng helps relieve physical or emotional stress and fatigue. It is stimulating and restorative, improving stamina and strength, alertness, and the ability to concentrate. It boosts metabolism and helps normalize body systems, including the production of glucose. It prevents fatigue during exercise.
- CAUTION
See General Guidelines on page 70.

DOSAGE
Depends on the grade of root. Choose a standardized product. Start with a low dose, increasing from 200 mg to 1,000 mg daily. The optimum dose is about 600 mg daily. To avoid overdose, take ginseng for two weeks on, then two weeks off.

BRAZILIAN GINSENG

Brazilian ginseng, also known as suma or pfaffia, is a rich source of amino acids, vitamins, minerals, and plant hormones that increase the uptake and use of oxygen in body cells. Unrelated to Chinese

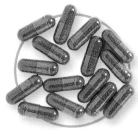

ginseng, pfaffia has similar adaptogenic properties, boosting physical, mental, and sexual energy. It enhances well-being by increasing resistance to stress and illness while improving the quality of sleep and helping the body overcome fatigue. In Brazil, it is regarded as a cure-all and is called *para todo* – "for everything."

Because of ginseng's beneficial effects on female hormonal balance, it is widely used by women whose energy is reduced before a period or during menopause. It is a natural alternative to HRT.

- **CAUTION**
See General Guidelines on page 70.

DOSAGE

Take 500–1,000 mg daily. Extracts standardized to contain 5 percent ecdysterones, a key constituent.

SIBERIAN GINSENG

Siberian ginseng is also an adaptogen, boosting physical and mental energy, especially under stress. It increases stamina and strength, particularly during or after illness. It is nonstimulating and is widely used by Russian athletes in training since it significantly improves performance and reaction times by decreasing lactic-acid buildup in muscles. It increases glycogen storage by up to 80 percent and maximizes oxygen usage. It also speeds up red blood cell production. It helps prolong sleep, normalizes glucose levels and blood pressure, and increases resistance to infection. It

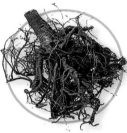

is widely used to boost the depleted energy levels associated with jet lag.

Siberian ginseng has similar actions to Korean ginseng but is not a stimulant. Those who find Korean ginseng too strong may find Siberian more suitable, especially if they suffer from anxiety.

- **CAUTION**
Do not take this herb while pregnant or breast-feeding. See General Guidelines on page 70.

DOSAGE

Take 250 mg–2 g daily. Extracts standardized to contain at least 1 percent eleutherosides, a key constituent. Start with a low dose and increase gradually. Take for two to three months on and one off.

GINKGO

Ginkgo improves memory and alertness by increasing peripheral blood supply as well as that to the brain. It boosts sexual energy by

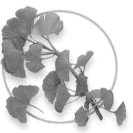

improving blood flow to the genitalia. It strengthens and maintains an erection, even in those with erectile difficulties. Among 50 men who took ginkgo for nine months, those who before had relied on drugs to get an erection regained their natural potency.

- **CAUTION**
Do not take ginkgo if on long-term blood-thinning medication. See General Guidelines on page 70.

DOSAGE

Take 40–60 mg three times daily. Extracts standardized to contain at least 24 percent ginkgolides, the key constituent.

GOTU KOLA

Gotu kola is one of the most important herbs in Ayurvedic medicine, in which it is known as brahmi. It is widely taken to increase physical and mental energy levels, improve memory and concentration, and relieve anxiety. It is reputed to increase longevity and hence it is known as the fountain of youth.

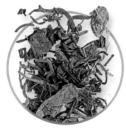

• CAUTION
High doses may cause headaches and be calming rather than energizing. See General Guidelines on page 70.

DOSAGE
Take 60–120 mg daily of extracts standardized to contain 40 percent asiaticoside (a key constituent) or 200 mg 2–3 times daily of 10 percent extracts.

GUARANA

Guarana is derived from a Brazilian bush known locally as "the food of the gods." The dried seeds contain a complex of natural stimulants, including guaranine – which resembles caffeine in its effects – and some substances similar to those in ginseng. Guarana increases physical, mental, and sexual energy, and is used to relieve fatigue and reduce the physical ill-effects of stress.

In one study it was found that, after taking guarana extracts for three

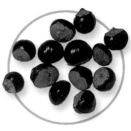

months, volunteers experienced a significant increase in energy levels and reacted better to stress. The caffeinelike effects of this herb are felt gradually so are less likely to produce the irritability, poor-quality sleep, and tremor associated with excessive caffeine intakes. Guarana therefore has a reputation for being a calming yet energizing stimulant. Some people, however, are sensitive to it and respond in the same way as they do to caffeine.

In Japan, guarana is used by long-distance drivers to stay awake. It is believed to have brought about a reduction in road traffic accidents caused by drivers falling asleep at the wheel. Guarana also helps prevent fatigue associated with jet lag if taken before, during, and after a long flight.

• CAUTION
In some sports guarana is included in the list of restricted substances. See General Guidelines on page 70.

DOSAGE
Take 1 g daily. A single dose provides an energy boost lasting up to six hours.

MACA

Maca is a Peruvian root vegetable, related to the potato, which is a good source of carbohydrate, amino acids, fatty acids, vitamins B, C, and E and

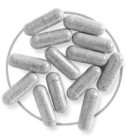

calcium, phosphorus, zinc, magnesium, copper, and iron. It is sometimes called Peruvian ginseng.

These tubers also contain a number of plant hormones that are known to increase energy levels. Maca is popular among athletes who want to increase their stamina. It also helps to relieve low-energy states associated with hormonal imbalance such as at the menopause.

• CAUTION
See General Guidelines on page 70.

DOSAGE
Take 1 g two to three times daily.

REISHI

Reishi is known to the Japanese as the "spiritual mushroom" and to the Chinese as the "mushroom of immortality." It has been used medicinally for more than 3,000 years and contains adenosine, a substance that is used in

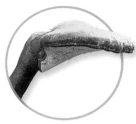

the body's energy storage and regulation system. Reishi is so effective at enhancing energy levels and improving sleep that, in one study, it was found to relieve weariness in 78 percent of the people taking it. It is a powerful adaptogen, tonic, and antioxidant that is used to promote vitality and longevity, strengthen many body systems, and increase intellectual capacity and memory.

Reishi has antiallergy, antibacterial, anticancer, antihistamine, antiviral, and anti-inflammatory properties that are being investigated further. The herb's effects are enhanced by the presence of vitamin C, which increases the absorption of reishi's active components.

• CAUTION

Check with a pharmacist or herbalist, especially if you take anticoagulants or drugs to reduce immunity or cholesterol levels. Avoid it while pregnant or breast-feeding, except under supervision. See General Guidelines on page 70.

DOSAGE
500 mg two to three times daily.

SCHISANDRA

Schisandra is a popular Chinese tonic herb that, like ginseng, has powerful adaptogenic properties to help you cope with stress.

Schisandra increases the uptake of oxygen in

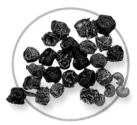

cells, increasing physical and sexual energy levels, improving mental acuity, and preventing physical and emotional fatigue. It also acts as an antioxidant and, overall, is regarded as a calming supplement that boosts liver function, enhances immunity and heart function, and eases allergic skin conditions. Furthermore, schisandra is a well-known sexual tonic, reputedly increasing the secretion of fluids.

DOSAGE
Take 250–500 mg one to three times daily for 100 days.

YERBA MATÉ

Yerba maté is rich in vitamins and minerals and is obtained from the leaves of a tree found in the Paraguayan rainforest. It contains xanthine alkaloids similar to those

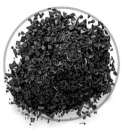

in coffee and guarana, and is used to increase mental alertness and acuity but without the side effects associated with caffeine. It is also thought to increase energy by making sleep more restful. Since they sleep better, some users find they need less sleep.

Yerba maté acts as an adaptogen by supporting adrenal gland function and helping the body cope with stress. It is a calming tonic, soothing anxiety and nervousness, improving concentration, and lifting mood. There may be other benefits such as better circulation and fewer allergic symptoms.

• CAUTION

Avoid taking yerba maté with food because its tannins may impair the absorption of nutrients. See General Guidelines on page 70.

DOSAGE
Drink two or three cups of yerba maté tea daily.

OTHER SUPPLEMENTS

Provide essential fatty acids ◆ Improve general well-being

◆ Boost immunity ◆ Balance hormones

EVENING PRIMROSE OIL

Oil from the seed of the evening primrose (EPO) is a rich source of essential fatty acid derivatives, such

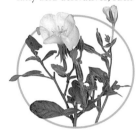

as gamma-linolenic acid (GLA), also known as gamolenic acid. GLA is metabolized to form hormonelike substances, prostaglandins. These are found in all body tissues and play a major role in regulating inflammation, blood clotting, hormonal balance, and immunity, all of which are closely linked to energy levels.

If there are insufficient essential fatty acids in the diet, the body makes do with the next best fatty acids available, such as those derived from saturated fats. This may cause a prostaglandin imbalance and, in turn, increase the risk of other imbalances, especially of sex hormones. Such imbalances are associated with dry and itchy skin, chronic inflammatory

diseases (rheumatoid arthritis, psoriasis, and eczema, for example) and gynecological problems, such as cyclical breast pain or premenstrual syndrome. A deficiency in essential fatty acids is also linked to fatigue. Research indicates that taking evening primrose oil supplements benefits as many as 80 percent of those people suffering from chronic fatigue.

As an oil, evening primrose is best taken at the same time as food to improve absorption. The action of the GLA is boosted by the presence of vitamin E, which also helps preserve it. Certain vitamins and minerals are also needed during the metabolism of essential fatty acids. These include vitamins B_3 (niacin), B_6 (pyridoxine), and C, magnesium, and zinc. Anyone taking evening primrose oil supplements should therefore ensure that their intake of these vitamins and minerals is adequate.

The only people for whom taking evening primrose oil is inadvisable are those who are allergic to the product and those suffering from a specific neurological disorder, temporal lobe epilepsy.

DOSAGE

Take 1 g of EPO daily for general health (equivalent to 80 mg of GLA). Take up to 3 g daily to treat hormone imbalance and fatigue. It may take about three months for the benefits to be appreciated.

ROYAL JELLY

Royal jelly is a milky-white substance secreted by the salivary glands of worker honeybees. It is a

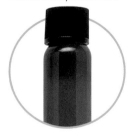

highly concentrated food and one of the richest natural sources of vitamin B_5 (pantothenic acid). It also contains other B vitamins as well as vitamins A, C, D, and E, 20 amino acids, essential fatty acids, minerals such as potassium, calcium, zinc, iron, and manganese, and acetylcholine – a neurotransmitter needed to pass messages from one nerve cell to another. Royal jelly is given by bees to all larvae for the first three days of their lives, and continued thereafter only for the larva destined to become queen bee. Royal jelly is such a nutritious and potent source of energy that the queen bee grows 50 percent larger than all other genetically identical female bees and lives nearly 40 times longer.

Royal jelly has been taken traditionally to boost energy levels and mental alertness and to combat stress, general fatigue, and insomnia. As a tonic, it increases well-being and vitality and improves the skin.

Royal jelly is best kept refrigerated and should be taken on an empty stomach. It needs to be blended with honey or freeze-dried to preserve its active ingredients.

• CAUTION
Do not take if you are allergic to bee products or you suffer from asthma or other allergies.

DOSAGE
Typically, take between 50 and 100 mg daily.

BEE POLLEN

When foraging for nectar in order to collect pollen, bees visit as many as 1,500 blossoms during their lifetime. Pollen is compressed into granules – known as bee pollen – for carrying back to the hive. Each one contains up to five million pollen grains. Granules are fed to young bees.

Bee pollen is rich in B-complex vitamins and essential fatty acids. It also contains 28 minerals and 22 amino acids as well as thousands of enzymes and coenzymes. It is widely taken as a general tonic and to improve energy levels. Bee pollen needs to be freeze-dried in order to preserve its active ingredients.

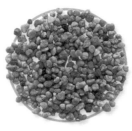

• CΛUTION
Do not take if you are allergic to bee products or you suffer from other allergic reactions.

DOSAGE
Start taking a few granules daily and, if you do not develop an allergic reaction (such as wheezing, a rash, a headache, or itchiness), increase the dose to 250 mg–2 g and take it for at least a month.

PROPOLIS

Propolis is a yellowy-brown sticky resin – also called bee glue – made by certain species of bees from wax mixed with the resinous sap of a number of trees, such as beech, birch, chestnut, and certain species of conifer. Bees use propolis as a

"cement" to repair cracks in the honeycombs and the hive. It is also placed around hive entrances to keep infections at bay.

Research shows that propolis has antiseptic

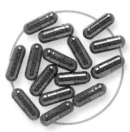

as well as antibacterial properties and is also a rich source of B vitamins and bioflavonoids, which help to improve the absorption and action of vitamin C. Propolis has been prescribed for more than 2,000 years for healing wounds and for boosting immunity and energy levels. Since it is not water soluble, it is extracted in alcohol and made into a tincture.

• CAUTION
Do not take if you are allergic to bee products or if you suffer from other allergic reactions. Propolis is known to cause a reaction in between one and seven percent of people using it, including contact dermatitis in those suffering from eczema.

DOSAGE
Take 250–500 mg daily. Propolis is available as chewing gum, chips, lozenges, and powdered in capsules.

ST. JOHN'S WORT

St. John's wort, otherwise know as hypericum, is a common shrubby plant with attractive yellow flowers found in many parts of the world. It was used to heal the wounds of Crusaders on the battlefield and has traditionally been given to people to drive away evil spirits as well as relieve physical ailments.

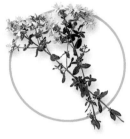

number of natural and effective antidepressant substances. These are known as hypericin, pseudohypericin, and hyperforin. They help maintain or even increase production of the brain's own feel-good chemical, serotonin. St. John's wort also helps relieve the effects of stress, especially longer-term nervous tension accompanied by mental as well as physical exhaustion. It also increases the body's nocturnal production of the hormone melatonin, the body's own natural sedative, thus improving the quality of sleep so that it is more restful.

St. John's wort is as effective in the treatment of mild to moderately severe depression as many of the conventionally prescribed antidepressants. In trials it has been shown to lift low spirits in at least 67 percent of those people suffering from mild to moderately severe depression. It is especially effective for treating seasonal affective disorder (SAD). People with this condition exhibit many of the symptoms of depression together with a lack of energy during the winter months. SAD is linked to reduced exposure to sunlight.

St. John's wort is also recommended for replenishing depleted energy levels (and raising low spirits and relieving anxiety and irritability) associated with hormone deficiencies in post-menopausal women and women who experience premenstrual syndrome. A pilot study involving about 20 women in their 20s and 30s with young children also found significant improvement in fatigue after they had taken St. John's wort.

- CAUTION

St. John's wort should not be mixed with certain conventional drugs. Check with your doctor.

DOSAGE

Take 300 mg three times a day. Extracts standardized to contain 0.3 percent hypericin, a key constituent. One-a-day formulas of St. John's wort are also available.

GENERAL GUIDELINES

Consider the following before taking herbal supplements. If in doubt, consult a practitioner.

- Always use products made by recognized, mainstream brands.
- Read manufacturers' recommendations carefully. You should avoid stimulants such as tea, coffee, or cola drinks, for example, when taking ginseng.
- The quantity of active ingredients in plants varies. Standardization ensures that every batch of a product provides the same degree of benefit.
- Seek advice about combining supplements. Vitamin C neutralizes ginseng, for example.
- If you are taking any prescribed medication, check with your doctor, pharmacist, or a qualified herbalist before taking supplements. St. John's wort cannot be mixed with certain drugs.
- Some supplements are not recommended for people with certain medical conditions. Ginseng should not be taken by those with high blood pressure or estrogen-dependent conditions such as breast cancer.
- Do not take any supplements while pregnant or breast-feeding unless under professional guidance.

EXERCISE FOR ENERGY

EXERCISE AND ENERGY PRODUCTION IN THE BODY ARE CLOSELY LINKED. THE MORE YOU EXERCISE, THE MORE ENERGY YOU PRODUCE, AND ULTIMATELY, THE MORE ENERGIZED YOU WILL FEEL. MANY FITNESS INSTRUCTORS RECOMMEND THAT YOU GET 30–40 MINUTES' EXERCISE BETWEEN THREE AND FIVE TIMES A WEEK.

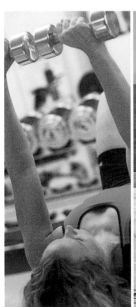

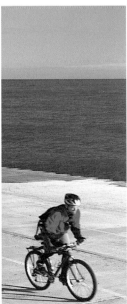

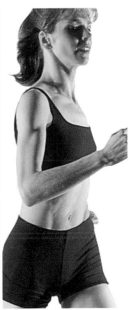

HOW EXERCISE BOOSTS ENERGY

Getting exercise regularly can significantly boost your physical, mental, and sexual energy levels so that you feel prepared to deal with anything that comes your way. It may even prolong your life.

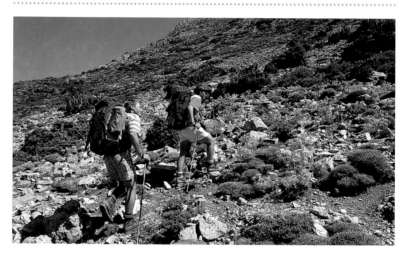

FUELING EXERCISE

During brisk exercise, your body's metabolic activity and the heat output within muscle cells increases to more than 20 times what it is when you are at rest. This in turn increases your overall metabolic rate by as much as a factor of 10 so that more energy is produced.

USING FAT

Fat stores are of little immediate use during exercise since they have to be mobilized and broken down into fatty acids before they can be used as a fuel, which takes too much time. During exercise, the muscles

Walking, especially up and down hills, is an excellent way of exercising, and provides an opportunity for escaping the stresses of life.

need a more immediate source of energy and take up glucose from the bloodstream and break down glycogen – a carbohydrate store found in muscle and liver cells. After exercise, muscle glycogen stores are quickly replenished when you eat carbohydrates. If these are in short supply, the body will break down protein to regenerate the glycogen instead. Eating just a small amount of glucose after exercise, therefore, can protect lean tissues from being broken down as emergency fuel.

This is why athletes often eat a banana, suck glucose tablets, or have a sports drink before, during, or after a performance.

GETTING ENERGIZED

If you are out of shape, starting an exercise program will leave you feeling temporarily fatigued, but this will pass and you will become more energized as you get fitter. This is because muscle glycogen stores are expandable. Muscles with a plentiful supply of glycogen can exercise for longer without tiring. In turn, this increases the bulk of muscle tissue and the amount of glycogen stored. An adult with a sedentary lifestyle has about 1 g of glycogen per 100 g of muscle, an athlete as much as 4 g per 100 g of muscle.

OTHER BENEFITS

Stamina increases with exercise as a result of greater circulation in the muscles and the improved efficiency of the heart and lungs, which allows more oxygen to get to where it is needed more quickly.

Exercise stimulates the release of feel-good substances in the brain known as endorphins. It may also reduce anxiety and tension and improve the quality of your sleep, thereby raising mental energy levels.

Interestingly, and contrary to popular belief, the expenditure of sexual energy can boost physical energy levels and physical performance. One Olympic middle-distance champion broke the world record an hour after making love.

Try to do at least 20–30 minutes of strenuous exercise five times a week. It is not necessary to overdo it, however. Heart specialists in Australia studied 500 men who either did light exercise on a bicycle, stair-stepper, and rowing machine with lots of rests, or who jogged or walked continuously for 30 minutes. After a year, both groups were equally fit in treadmill tests.

The more exercise you do, the more you will be able to do. As your fitness level improves, your muscles can exercise for longer without tiring.

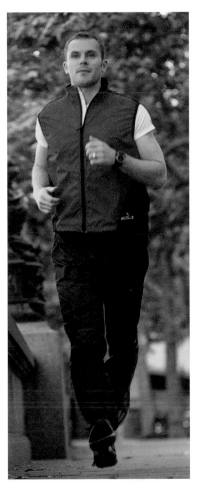

HOW MUCH EXERCISE?

If you can exercise fairly strenuously for 30–40 minutes at least three, but preferably five, times a week you will feel significantly more energized than if you remain largely inactive. You do not have to become an exercise fanatic, however. Activities such as home renovation, gardening, and dancing are just as effective as swimming or bicycling for heart health. Even a brisk walk to and from the grocery store or the office on a regular basis will keep you fit. Any activity that leaves you feeling warm and slightly out of breath is doing you good. And the half-hour's exercise does not have to be done all in one stretch either. You can divide it up into two or three 10- or 15-minute sessions throughout the day if you prefer.

CHOOSING AN ACTIVITY

If you prefer exercising alone, consider:

- Walking, especially power-walking or hill-walking
- Dog-walking
- Jogging
- Bicycling
- Swimming
- Home gym workout
- Weight-training
- Gardening
- Horseback riding
- In-line skating
- Ice-skating
- Trampolining
- Skipping
- Yoga
- T'ai chi

If you prefer companionable exercise, choose from:

- Dog-walking with friends
- Hiking
- Golf
- Bowling
- Table tennis
- Gym workout
- Aerobic workout or aquarobics
- Body conditioning class
- Dancing class, such as salsa, belly-dancing, hip hop, or jive
- Tennis
- Badminton
- Squash
- Team sport such as netball, volleyball, baseball, soccer, or hockey
- Strides (indoor jogging), spinning (indoor cycling to music), or crew class (indoor rowing)
- T'ai chi class
- Tae kwon do class

If you need motivation or direction, consider:

- Home exercise video
- One-to-one fitness program under the supervision of a personal trainer, either at home or in a gym
- Exercise class at a gym or sports center
- Fitness program organized by a sports club
- Kick-boxing or other martial-arts-based activity
- Circuit-training
- Park circuits
- Bootcamp workout
- Team sports
- Athletics
- Dance class
- Strides, spinning, or crew class
- Pilates
- Flexaball workout

WHAT DOES EXERCISING ACHIEVE?

Exercise improves strength (by building up muscle bulk), stamina (by increasing muscle energy stores), and suppleness (by improving the range of movement of joints and making ligaments and tendons more flexible). Different sports and activities have different effects on increasing your degrees of strength, stamina, and suppleness.

HEALTH BENEFITS OF DIFFERENT SPORTS

The following exercises have different effects:

| * | Slight effect | ** | Beneficial effect |
| *** | Very good effect | **** | Excellent effect |

Activity	Stamina	Strength	Suppleness
Judo/karate	*	*	**
Baseball	*	*	**
Golf	*	*	**
Yoga	*	*	***
Weight-training	*	****	**
Walking (hiking)	**	*	*
Softball	**	**	*
Downhill skiing	**	**	**
Tennis	**	**	***
Badminton	**	**	***
Power- or hill-walking	***	**	*
Rowing	***	**	*
Skipping	***	**	**
Aerobics	***	**	***
Squash	***	**	***
Athletics	***	**	**
Circuit-training	***	***	***
Soccer	***	***	***
Jogging	****	**	**
Bicycling	****	***	**
Strong swimming	****	****	****

GETTING STARTED

If you have not exercised for years and are relatively unfit, you should consult your doctor before doing anything. Anyone who has joint problems, for example, will be advised to try a nonweight-bearing exercise such as swimming or cycling. To get fit effectively and safely, do not launch straight into a strenuous fitness program. Start off slowly and exercise regularly for about 20 minutes three times a week. Once your fitness level increases, you can do more exercise.

Whatever your fitness level, exercise should be strenuous enough to raise your pulse to about 100 beats a minute, to work up a slight sweat, and to leave you feeling slightly breathless (but still able to hold a conversation). At the end of a session you should feel invigorated and energized, not exhausted.

Dog-walking is a great way of staying in shape, both for you and your dog. If you do not have a dog, get together with friends while they walk theirs and you will have companionship as well as someone to motivate you.

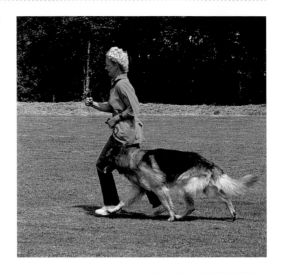

EXERCISING SAFELY

- Always warm up first with a few simple bends and stretches and some brisk walking or a gentle jog
- Cool down afterward by walking around for a few minutes and stretching out
- Wear loose clothing and suitable footwear specifically designed for the activity; use any recommended safety equipment.
- Try to exercise away from traffic and, if you are out at night, wear reflective colors and fluorescent strips
- If you are under a doctor's care for any medical condition – especially a heart problem – or if you are taking medication, seek medical advice before starting a physical exercise program

HOW TO GET MORE EXERCISE

- Take up an active hobby, such as dancing, in-line or ice skating, swimming, yoga, t'ai chi, or bicycling
- Borrow a dog and take it for regular walks
- Walk up the stairs instead of using the elevator or an escalator
- Walk or bicycle reasonable distances instead of using the car
- Walk around the block in your lunch hour
- If you cannot go out, try walking briskly up- and downstairs a few times a day
- Reintroduce the traditional habit of a family walk after Sunday lunch
- Get off the bus or subway one stop earlier than usual and walk the rest of the way
- Get up an hour earlier than usual and go for a walk, bicycle, do some gardening, walk to the store to buy a newspaper, or visit the gym
- Buy a home exercise machine and use it while watching or listening to the evening news
- Spend less time watching television or sitting in front of a computer and more time working in the garden or around the house; listen to music or the radio if you like background noise
- If you dislike exercise, put more effort into home renovation or gardening

IMPROVING MENTAL ENERGY

A NUMBER OF TECHNIQUES MAY HELP IMPROVE YOUR MENTAL ENERGY LEVELS WHEN YOU ARE FEELING JADED. THESE VARY FROM INHALING INVIGORATING AROMATHERAPY OILS AND VISUALIZING VIBRANT COLORS TO TAKING AN ENERGIZING SUPPLEMENT SUCH AS GUARANA OR MAINTAINING AN ENERGY-GIVING YOGA POSTURE.

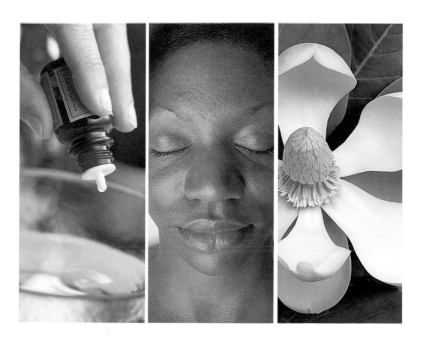

INCREASING MENTAL ENERGY

Nutrient supplements, mental and spiritual disciplines, and healing techniques really can improve your memory, increase the recall of new information, and improve overall concentration and mental performance.

TAKING SUPPLEMENTS

Taking a good multinutrient supplement each day acts as a safety net, preventing deficiencies in vitamins or minerals that may affect your mental energy levels. Thiamine and other B-group vitamins and potassium, calcium, magnesium, iron, and zinc are vitally important for mental energy and good memory function.

If your mental energy levels are depleted, trials have shown that *Ginkgo biloba* extracts significantly improve short-term working memory within just two days – probably by improving blood circulation to the brain. Another supplement, phosphatidyl serine, has also been shown to improve all cognitive functions, including learning, recall,

recognition, and concentration by providing the nutrients needed to synthesize brain neurotransmitters. It seems to work by increasing the metabolism of glucose within brain cells and speeding up transmission of messages from one neuron (nerve cell) to another. Phosphatidylserine and ginkgo may be taken together. Fish has traditionally been known as a brain food, and researchers have found that in fact it contains phosphatidyl choline, a substance needed to manufacture the neurotransmitter, acetylcholine.

Essential oils and other natural remedies can stimulate the mind generally or address a specific mental state.

COMPLEMENTARY THERAPIES

The holistic nature of many complementary therapies means that mental energy levels are assessed as an integral part of the treatment, whatever your condition.

Traditional Eastern therapies such as acupuncture, reflexology, and shiatsu are believed to stimulate the flow of "life energy" to the brain and all parts of the body.

Other touch therapies involve the application of presssure or gentle manipulation. Craniosacral therapy, for example, involves the laying on of hands, mainly over the skull and lower spine. Experienced therapists assess the flow of cerebro-spinal fluid (known as the cranial rhythmic impulse) and "listen" to the inner movements and tensions of the body. This is believed to release inner energy, relieve tension, and boost mental energy levels.

Homeopathy is based on the belief that natural substances boost the body's own healing powers to relieve the symptoms of illness. A homeopathic practitioner assesses your constitutional type, personality, lifestyle, and likes and dislikes as well as your physical symptoms. Some remedies are selected according to emotional traits displayed such as anger, timidity, or anxiety, and these are particularly useful in treating ailments that are accompanied by low mental energy levels.

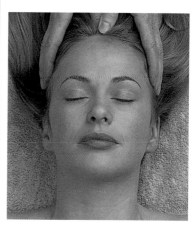

Most people undergoing craniosacral therapy feel deeply relaxed during a treatment. It is especially good for relieving tension headaches.

AROMATHERAPY

Essential oils have a beneficial effect on the mind, clarifying thoughts and improving alertness. Place a few drops of the appropriate oil on a handkerchief and inhale.

MENTALLY UPLIFTING ESSENTIAL OILS

Type of oil	Effect
◆ Basil	for clarity
◆ Bergamot	for extra confidence
◆ Rosemary	for improved memory
◆ Lemon	for better concentration
◆ Ginger	to help overcome forgetfulness
◆ Cardamom	for clarity
◆ Coriander	for improved memory
◆ Black pepper	to overcome emotional blocks and mental exhaustion
◆ Peppermint	for physical and mental uplift

INSTANT MENTAL ENERGIZERS

Whenever you need a quick mental energy recharge, try
one of these ten energy-boosting techniques for
an instant pick-me-up. You will feel more alert
and your concentration will be greater as a result.

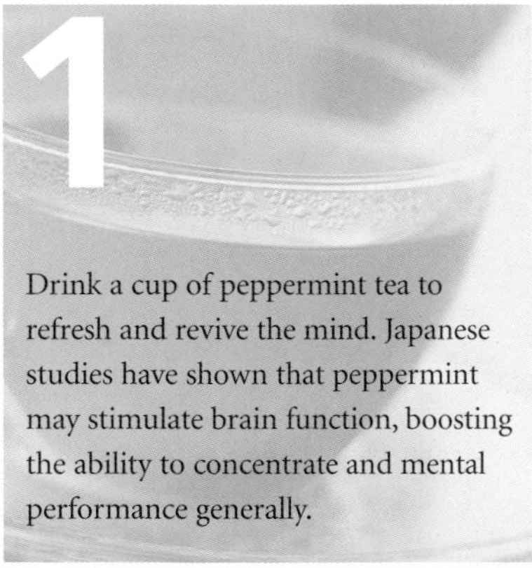

1

Drink a cup of peppermint tea to refresh and revive the mind. Japanese studies have shown that peppermint may stimulate brain function, boosting the ability to concentrate and mental performance generally.

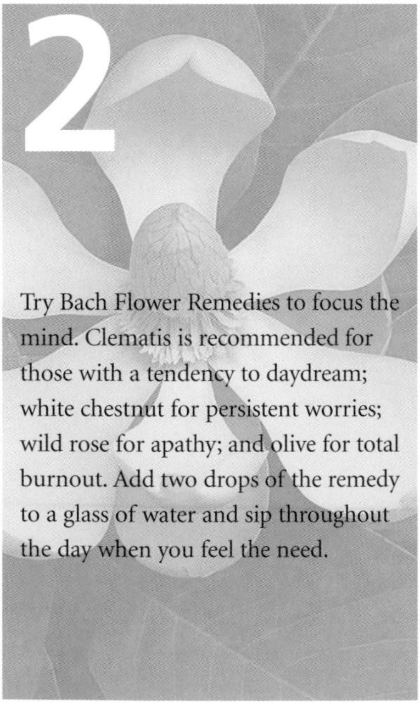

2

Try Bach Flower Remedies to focus the mind. Clematis is recommended for those with a tendency to daydream; white chestnut for persistent worries; wild rose for apathy; and olive for total burnout. Add two drops of the remedy to a glass of water and sip throughout the day when you feel the need.

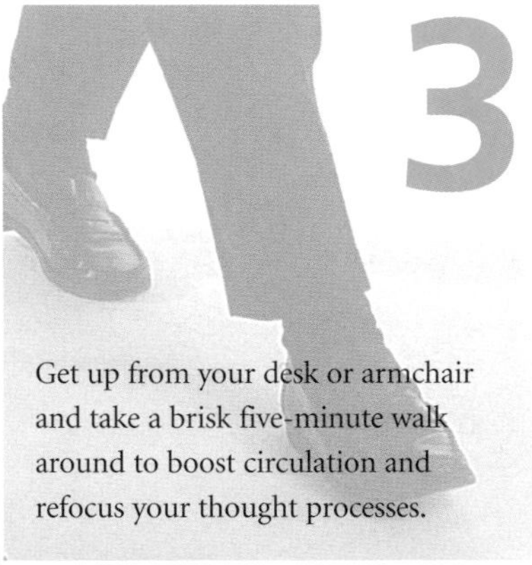

3

Get up from your desk or armchair and take a brisk five-minute walk around to boost circulation and refocus your thought processes.

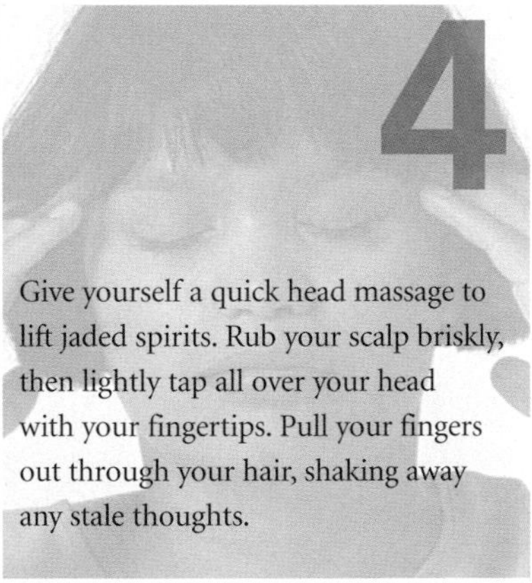

4

Give yourself a quick head massage to lift jaded spirits. Rub your scalp briskly, then lightly tap all over your head with your fingertips. Pull your fingers out through your hair, shaking away any stale thoughts.

5

Eat a handful of Brazil nuts. These are a good source of magnesium, which helps clear a muddled head and lift a bad mood. They also contain the antioxidant mineral selenium.

6

Visualize an uplifting color. Orange is good for lethargy or fatigue. Sit or lie comfortably, eyes closed, and imagine the color seeping up through your fingers and toes to suffuse every part of the body as you inhale deeply. Pause and feel your body tingling and warming. Exhale and imagine the color evaporating with your breath, freeing up all your mental blocks. Open your eyes and feel awake.

7

Inhale an essential oil, which will travel within seconds to the limbic system in the brain, the part associated with mood and emotions. Choose bergamot to revive, lemongrass to counter sluggishness, orange to lighten mood, and rose to increase alertness; or blend a combination of oils. Add five drops of essential oil to 10 ml sweet almond carrier oil and use in a vaporizer, or drip the oil onto a handkerchief and inhale as necessary.

Yoga postures known as inversions send a fresh supply of blood to the brain, with revitalizing effects. Beginners should try *halasana* (the plow). See page 92 for step-by-step instructions. More advanced students of yoga may like to opt for *salamba sirshasana* (the headstand), which requires a greater level of ability.

8

Absorb vitality from your crown chakra, regarded as one of the body's most important sites of energy in Ayurveda. Envision a sphere of light pulsating and spinning just above your head. Breathe in its energy for a few moments, absorbing its ability to enhance brain power, increase open-mindedness, and counter cynicism. If you are alone, try saying "eeee" to yourself as you do this, which is claimed to help rebalance this chakra.

9

10

Stimulate key acupoints to tap into the body's energy channels and encourage the circulation of *qi* or life energy. For relief from pain in the head and face caused by mental stress, press the area where your thumb and forefinger meet between the thumb and forefinger of the other hand. Hold this for five seconds, then release.

MEDITATION

Induces profound relaxation ◆ Reduces stress ◆ Relieves
fatigue ◆ Increases general sense of well-being

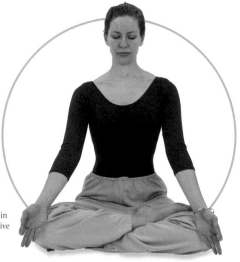

MEDITATION
Sit comfortably and in
a way that is conducive
to calm thoughts.

KEY PRINCIPLES

Meditation is an ancient
technique used widely in
both Eastern and Western
cultures to relax physically
and boost mental energy.
It uses the power of the
mind to clear the head
of all thought, calm the
body, and achieve a state
of heightened mental or
spiritual awareness. This
is achieved by focusing on
an object or vision.

ENTERING A
MEDITATIVE STATE

There are several things
you can focus on: your
breathing; a universal
mystical sound such as
"om"; a mandala (an
intricate, often geometric
design or symbol); a
mantra (a sacred word or
phrase or one that is of

significance to you); or a
flickering candle flame or
an object such as a flower.
Alternatively, you can use
a repetitive action, such
as moving beads along a
thread, in order to focus.

To guide yourself into
a meditative state using
one of these, imagine
your body becoming
increasingly weightless,
bathed in healing energy.

A popular, accessible
meditative technique
is Transcendental
Meditation (TM), which
uses Sanskrit mantras to
help you still your mind
and find a deeper level of
consciousness. This is
intended to be practiced
for 15 to 20 minutes twice
a day, and is designed to
slot into any lifestyle –
however busy. TM helps

you achieve a state of
deep relaxation while
staying fully alert. It leaves
you feeling mentally and
physically energized,
with improved clarity of
thought, ready to face the
challenges of the day.

On coming out of a
meditative state, it is
important to sit or lie
quietly for a few moments
in order to collect your
thoughts and come back
fully into the real world.

HOW TO LEARN

It is advisable to learn
meditation under
the guidance of an
instructor, but you
can, with motivation
and self-discipline,
teach yourself from
a book or video.

VISUALIZATION

Reduces stress ◆ Encourages the body's self-healing

processes ◆ Increases general sense of well-being

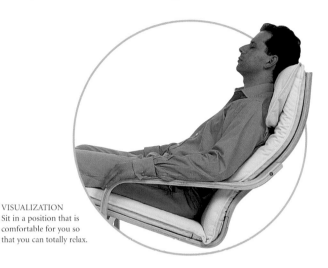

VISUALIZATION
Sit in a position that is
comfortable for you so
that you can totally relax.

KEY PRINCIPLES

Visualization is similar to meditation but instead of emptying the mind of thought, you use your imagination to go on a journey to a quiet place where you will become energized. It uses the power of suggestion and positive thinking to transform a desirable goal – whether it be reducing stress, fighting an illness, or achieving success – into reality. Visualization helps you become totally relaxed physically and well-balanced emotionally.

A VISUALIZATION EXERCISE

Sit or lie, whichever is most comfortable for you, in a quiet, darkened or candlelit room. A typical flight of imagination might take you through a door onto a tranquil beach beside a calm, azure blue sea. Waves gently lap at the edge of golden sands. Aromatic tropical flowers scent the air with vanilla, jasmine, and rose as warm evening sunlight filters down through coconut palms. You feel a slight breeze against your skin and you can hear cicadas starting to chirp in the foliage. Use your senses to explore the colors, sounds, smells, and other sensations in this secret world as you drift deeper and deeper into a calm, relaxed, meditative state.

Boost your energy levels further by thinking about energizing sunlight suffusing your body. When it is time to bring your inner journey to an end, picture yourself walking back through the door and closing it behind you before opening your eyes, stretching, and rejoining the present.

If you visualize in this way just before you go to sleep, your subconscious mind will dwell on the goal you are striving for and may well help make it more achievable.

HOW TO LEARN

Visualization may be guided by a therapist or a relaxation tape so that your thoughts are led, or you can allow them to wander freely.

POSITIVE THINKING

Reduces stress ◆ Improves self-esteem ◆ Reenergizes
mind and body ◆ Helps maintain general good health

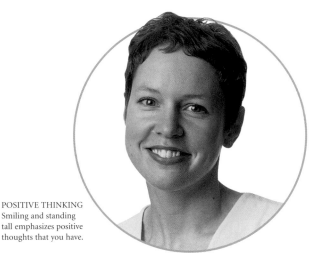

POSITIVE THINKING
Smiling and standing
tall emphasizes positive
thoughts that you have.

KEY PRINCIPLES

Positive thinking is a powerful force that can be harnessed and used to boost flagging energy levels and even to fight illness. By thinking positively, you can help change negative patterns of subconscious thought, which drain you of a lot of energy, into positive ones to help you banish fatigue.

MAKING STATEMENTS

The power of positive thinking should not be underestimated. If you have negative thoughts about yourself, your self-esteem and energy levels will suffer. To help you feel more positive, write down ten qualities you like about yourself, such

as "I have a good sense of humor"; "I am loyal"; "I am intelligent"; or "I am willing to help others."

These are exceptional qualities that no one can take away from you. Write out the list again, but this time on a small piece of paper, putting the items in order of importance to you. Place this second list in your wallet or purse and the next time your self-esteem suffers a knock or you feel that you are incapable of doing the task in front of you, read the list before you are consumed by negativity.

Next, write down a list of all the negative feelings you have about yourself. Change them around so that they become positive statements. For example,

"I am not an important person" becomes "I am just as important as everyone else"; and "This task is too difficult" becomes "I am totally capable of doing this."

The more you reread these affirmations, the more they will become imprinted on your belief systems, and gradually your levels of emotional energy will increase.

HOW TO LEARN

Learning methods of reinforcing positive thinking is possible on your own, or you can consult a practitioner trained in techniques of auto-suggestion, hypnosis, or visualization.

BREATHING TECHNIQUES

Induces relaxation and reduces stress ◆ Ensures a good

oxygen supply ◆ Reenergizes body and mind

BREATHING
Feel how your chest and
ribcage move as you
inhale and exhale.

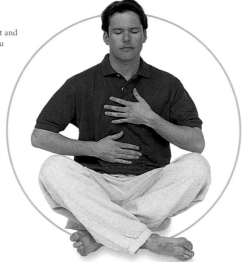

KEY PRINCIPLES

Oxygen is vital for energy production, and the way you breathe affects your energy levels. If your breathing is too shallow, you will not obtain all the oxygen you need for the optimum production of energy. If you over-breathe, however, you may exhale too much carbon dioxide and the blood will become too alkaline. This is known as hyperventilation and may result in weakness, pins and needles, shakiness, fatigue, panic, and anxiety.

BREATHING EASY

To help you recognize what normal breathing feels like, lie comfortably and rest your hands on your upper chest. Be aware of the rise and fall of your chest as you inhale and exhale. Imagine the flame of a candle just in front of your face and breathe gently so that it hardly flickers. Then place your hands on your lower ribcage so your fingertips just touch when you have exhaled. Now, as you gently breathe in, notice how your ribcage moves upward and outward.

Be aware of your breathing on a day-to-day basis while you are doing different activities, and monitor any changes. It is easy for bad breathing habits to be reestablished. Try to develop a slow, calm breathing rhythm that has a slight pause after each exhalation.

When you have inhaled as much as you comfortably can, immediately start to exhale and empty your lungs of as much air as possible. It will help you establish a breathing rhythm if you slowly count up to three while inhaling and counting up to four when exhaling.

HOW TO LEARN

You can teach yourself, and simple techniques are taught in clinics and hospitals. Many practitioners use breathing techniques to therapeutic effect, as do teachers of movement therapies such as yoga, pilates, t'ai chi, and qigong.

BACH FLOWER REMEDIES

Dispel negative, energy-sapping emotions ◆ Relieve the physical symptoms of emotional disorders

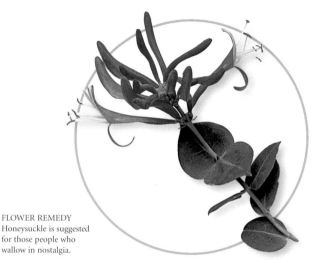

FLOWER REMEDY
Honeysuckle is suggested
for those people who
wallow in nostalgia.

KEY PRINCIPLES

Flower remedies are homeopathic preparations in which flower essences are preserved in grape alcohol (brandy). They are designed to relieve a variety of emotional states associated with low levels of energy.

Edward Bach devised his flower remedies in the early 20th century. He believed that physical symptoms such as fatigue were due to underlying emotional stresses. He classified emotional problems into seven major groups, which were further subdivided into 38 negative or harmful states of mind. He then identified a flower essence for each state to restore emotional balance. Some often-used remedies are listed opposite.

Bach Flower Remedies are prepared either by infusion or boiling. In the first case, flower heads are placed on the surface of pure springwater and left to infuse in sunlight. The infused water is preserved in grape alcohol, creating a mother tincture, which is diluted to make the remedies. Alternatively, short twigs bearing flowers or catkins are boiled in springwater for 30 minutes. The solution is cooled and preserved in alcohol. Flower remedies are available over-the-counter in most good pharmacies and health food outlets. Place two drops on the tongue or add them to a glass of water and sip until the feelings have passed. Remedies may be mixed.

HOW TO USE

Flower remedies were intended to be self-prescribed, so you can assess your emotional state and choose a remedy accordingly. Some complementary practitioners, such as homeopaths or aromatherapists, may prescribe them.

FOR FEAR

Rock rose	Extreme terror, panic, fright, nightmares
Mimulus	Known fears (such as phobias), timidity, shyness
Cherry plum	Fear of uncontrollable rage, causing harm
Aspen	Vague fear and anxiety, foreboding, apprehension
Red chestnut	Excessive fear or overconcern for others

FOR UNCERTAINTY AND INDECISION

Cerato	Doubt about ability to judge situations
Scleranthus	Indecision, mood swings
Gentian	Hesitancy, despondency, self-doubt
Gorse	Despair, hopelessness, futility
Hornbeam	Inability to face the day, procrastination

FOR INSUFFICIENT INTEREST IN PRESENT CIRCUMSTANCES

Clematis	Escapism, lack of concentration, daydreaming
Honeysuckle	Nostalgia, homesickness, living in the past
Wild rose	Apathy, resignation to circumstances
Olive	Total exhaustion, weariness, sapped vitality

FOR OVERSENSITIVITY TO INFLUENCES AND IDEAS

Agrimony	Reluctance to burden others, concealing problems
Centaury	Inability to say no, anxiety to please
Walnut	Instability of emotions during transition
Holly	Negative feelings such as envy, suspicion, revenge, hatred

FOR LONELINESS

Water violet	Desire to be alone, aloofness, reluctance to get involved in others' problems
Impatiens	Speed in thought and action but with irritability or impatience of those who are slower
Heather	Excessive talkativeness, desire for companionship

FOR DESPONDENCY OR DESPAIR

Larch	Lack of self-confidence, anticipation of failure
Pine	Self-reproach, guilt, dissatisfaction with actions
Elm	Overstretching, overburdening of responsibility
Sweet chestnut	Inability to endure, deep despair, great anguish

FOR OVERCONCERN FOR THE WELFARE OF OTHERS

Chicory	Reluctance to let family and friends go
Vervain	Strong opinions, deep sense of injustice
Vine	Strong will, ruthlessness, inflexibility
Beech	Intolerance, desire for perfection, overcriticism

MASSAGE

Deeply relaxing ◆ Boosts the body's self-healing
mechanisms ◆ Maintains good health and well-being

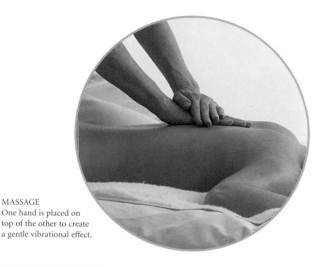

MASSAGE
One hand is placed on
top of the other to create
a gentle vibrational effect.

KEY PRINCIPLES

Massage is one of the oldest healing techniques and forms a part of many complementary therapies. It stimulates soft tissue, encouraging drainage and the removal of toxins, promotes relaxation, and improves the quality of sleep, raising physical and mental energy levels. Massage lotions and oils containing energizing aromatherapy oil blends are widely available and increase the therapeutic value of a massage.

THE ART OF GENTLE MASSAGE

A variety of strokes are used – including stroking, drumming, rubbing, kneading, and wringing – and different levels of pressure can be applied. A warm, quiet environment, with soft candlelight and relaxing music playing softly help to set the scene. The person being massaged should lie on a firm surface and be covered with a towel or sheet. Massage oil or lotion should be warmed.

Each area of the body in turn is uncovered, massaged, then covered again. A massage should begin with long, simple strokes that follow body contours and warm the skin. Movements are flowing and rhythmic, with one hand in contact with the body at all times. Strokes move toward the heart as a general rule.

The pressure and length of strokes can be varied. Firm movements can be alternated with light, feathery ones. If a muscle seems knotted or tense, gentle kneading movements concentrated on the spot will smooth away tension or pain.

HOW TO LEARN

A variety of massage techniques have been incorporated into complementary treatments, such as aromatherapy. It is possible to massage yourself – though the benefits are unlikely to be as intense as being treated by a masseuse – but advanced techniques are best left to those trained to use them.

INCREASING SPIRITUAL ENERGY

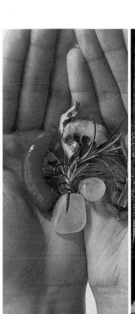

SOME THERAPIES PRESUPPOSE THE EXISTENCE OF AN EXTERNAL SPIRITUAL ENERGY – OFTEN DESCRIBED AS UNIVERSAL ENERGY. THESE INCLUDE SPIRITUAL HEALING AND REIKI. OTHERS DRAW ON YOUR INNER RESERVES OF SPIRITUAL ENERGY WITH THE AIM OF STRENGTHENING IT (FOR EXAMPLE, YOGA), WHILE YET OTHER THERAPIES, SUCH AS CRYSTAL OR COLOR THERAPY, RELY ON ELECTROMAGNETIC RESONANCE TO BOOST YOUR ENERGY LEVELS.

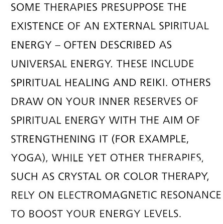
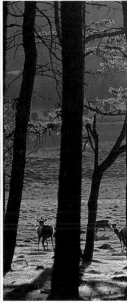
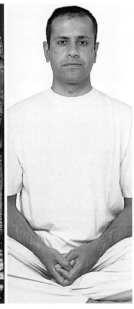

TAPPING IN TO SPIRITUAL ENERGY

In holistic medicine, spiritual energy is viewed as having equal, if not greater, importance to physical and mental energy. A number of therapies aim to help you connect more deeply with your inner self.

SPIRITUAL WELL-BEING

How much spiritual energy we have – the way in which and the extent to which we respond to spiritual matters – is dependent on a complex network of interwoven factors. Our belief systems, how fit and healthy we are, the quality of our home and working lives, our relationships, how we react to stress, and our experience of traumatic life events like divorce or death are but a few.

LOCATING ENERGY WITHIN

Increasing spiritual energy is a personal project that can be tackled on a number of levels. A hobby such as voluntary work – visiting the elderly or feeding the homeless – can be spiritually rewarding, and activities such as gardening or hiking open your mind as well your eyes to the beauty of the natural world.

Many movement therapies, as well as being of physical benefit, expand the mind in a spiritual sense.

Art, dance, music, and movement therapies are regarded as spiritual activities. They allow you to express inner feelings that otherwise might be difficult to express. Movement therapy can be unstructured, so you play music and move in whatever way feels right at the time, or it can be structured, so you repeat set movements, as in t'ai chi or qigong. Set pieces can be individually tailored, however, to allow your inner spirit to express itself.

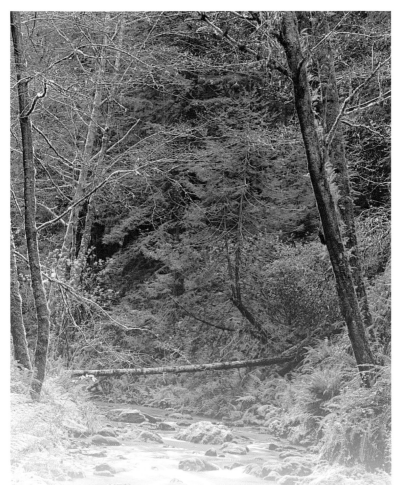

HEALING TECHNIQUES

A number of techniques help you locate and access spiritual energy within you. The Chinese believe that your constitutional essence, or *jing*, is boosted by activating the *tan tien*, the area just below your navel where *jing* is located. The technique for doing this is the inner smile. Think about something that makes you smile but inwardly, not visibly. Imagine feelings of strength, energy, and harmony spreading through your body and concentrating where *jing* is based in the *tan tien*.

Appreciating scenes of natural beauty may induce tranquility and inner peace and will ultimately be spiritually uplifting.

Another method is hypnotherapy, whereby suggestions are made while you are in a profoundly relaxed state to help you replace old, unwanted behavior patterns or beliefs with positive new messages.

Spiritual healing techniques are believed to channel universal energy into those needing a spiritual boost. You do not need a particular faith, just an open mind to the possibility that spiritual energy can be of help.

YOGA

Complete system for physical, mental, and spiritual
well-being ◆ Revitalizes all body systems

YOGA
Halasana, or the plow,
is a revitalizing
inversion posture.

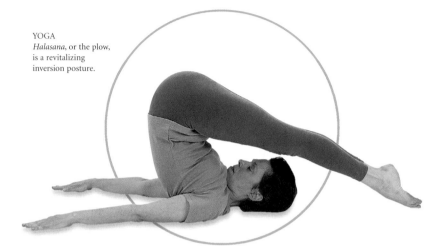

KEY PRINCIPLES

This mystical, spiritual movement therapy uses postures (*asanas*), breathing techniques (*pranayama*), and meditation (*dhyana*) to encourage union between mind, body, and spirit. Rigorous practice achieves the ultimate goal of self-enlightenment. Postures known as inversions have a particularly revitalizing effect on physical, mental, and spiritual energy. Beginners should try *halasana*, the plow, while advanced students may opt for *salamba sirsasana*, the headstand.

HALASANA

You are recommended to go into the half or full shoulderstand first. Lie on your back, with legs outstretched, feet together, and arms by your sides (palms down). Exhale and lift your legs into the air, bringing the hips off the floor and supporting them with your hands. Hold this position for a few breaths. Slowly lower your feet to the floor behind your head, keeping your feet together and the toes pointed. Release your hands from supporting the back and lower the arms so they are pointing in the opposite direction to the legs. Keep the neck relaxed and do not press your chin into your chest. Look toward the heart chakra and hold for as long as is comfortable before carefully coming out of the position.

• CAUTION
Only do this if you have been instructed properly. Do not do it if you are pregnant, menstruating, or obese, or if you have high blood pressure or other high risk factors for heart disease or stroke, a detached retina, neck or back problems, or if you have had recent surgery.

HOW TO LEARN
It is possible to teach yourself yoga from the many books or tapes available, but many people find it helpful to learn under the guidance of a teacher who can advise you about breathing and appropriate postures.

HYPNOTHERAPY

Counteracts energy-draining thoughts and behavior
◆ Relieves stress ◆ Induces relaxation

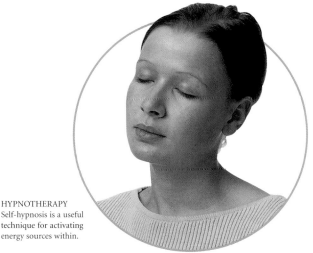

HYPNOTHERAPY
Self-hypnosis is a useful
technique for activating
energy sources within.

KEY PRINCIPLES

The subconscious mind responds to messages you send it to "reprogram" behavior and thought processes. Hypnotherapy is most commonly used to strengthen the resolve and overcome addictive or obsessive behavior and phobias. It is useful for overcoming a lack of confidence, releasing blocked creativity, and helping to control pain or emotional distress.

DO IT YOURSELF

Relax in a warm, quiet, dimly lit room where you will not be disturbed. Sit or lie comfortably with hands by your sides and feet apart. Roll your eyes upward and fix your eyes on a spot (imagined or real) on the ceiling. Inhale as deeply as you can. Hold the breath during a slow count to ten, then exhale as much as possible while saying quietly to yourself "relax." Repeat three times, closing your eyes during the last exhalation.

Now imagine your body is weightless and you are slowly floating down a flight of ten stairs, counting backward from five very slowly. Once you are at the bottom of the stairs, focus on the change you want to make in yourself, for example, "I am full of energy" or "I am self-confident." Always use the present tense since the subconscious mind responds best to this. Imagine yourself in your new, more energized state,

and keep repeating the positive statement.

After ten minutes of visualization, tell yourself that on the count of five you will slowly float back up the staircase, open your eyes, and feel refreshed and revitalized.

Try to practice self-hypnosis every day. It is an excellent technique for increasing energy levels and helping you achieve a general state of relaxation.

HOW TO LEARN
You can learn self-hypnosis from a book or tape, but it is best to consult a qualified hypnotherapist first. A few sessions might be helpful prior to a self-help program.

AROMATHERAPY

Promotes general well-being ◆ Relieves energy-sapping
conditions ◆ Induces relaxation

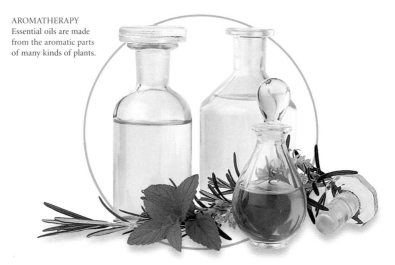

AROMATHERAPY
Essential oils are made
from the aromatic parts
of many kinds of plants.

KEY PRINCIPLES

Aromatherapy uses
aromatic essential oils
obtained from the flowers,
seeds, leaves, stems, bark,
or roots of plants and
trees. These oils contain
many active ingredients
in a highly concentrated
and potent form which,
because the oils are
volatile, readily evaporate
to release their powerful
scents. Oils that come
into contact with the skin
are absorbed and may
have therapeutic effects.

CHOOSING OILS

Energizing oils used for
boosting physical, mental,
or sexual energy include
angelica, benzoin, black
pepper, cardamom, lemon,
orange, peppermint, pine,
rosemary, rosewood, and
sandalwood. Oils may be
inhaled, massaged into
the skin, added to a bath,
rubbed into the skin in
the shower, or added to a
pot pourri, sprayed into
the air, or heated in order
to perfume and energize
the atmosphere.

Choose oils carefully,
preferably under the
guidance of a qualified
aromatherapist, and
follow manufacturers'
instructions with care.
Use natural rather than
synthetic oils. These have
a fuller, sweeter aroma
that provides a greater
therapeutic benefit. Also,
make sure you select 100
percent pure oils. These
are often more expensive
but have a greater effect;
they are not blended with
alcohol or other additives.

• **CAUTION**
**Do not use essential oils
if you are pregnant or
have a medical condition
such as high blood
pressure or epilepsy,
unless under supervision.**

HOW TO USE

Essential oil should
always be diluted in
a carrier oil, such as
almond, jojoba, or
wheat germ, before it
is massaged into the
skin or added to
bathwater because it
may irritate the skin.
Add no more than
1 drop of essential
oil to 24 drops of
carrier oil (10 ml or
2 tsp of carrier oil to
at most 5 drops of
essential oil).

CRYSTAL THERAPY

Encourages the body's own healing processes

◆ Balances and boosts energy levels

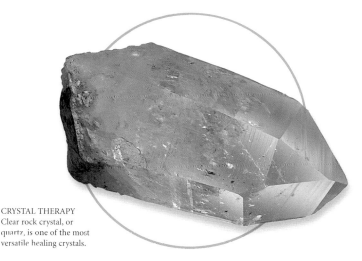

CRYSTAL THERAPY
Clear rock crystal, or
quartz, is one of the most
versatile healing crystals.

KEY PRINCIPLES

Crystal therapy aims to harness the energy within the rocks in the Earth's crust, some of which are more than 40 million years old. Crystals are believed to be tuned into the Earth's magnetic field, to resonate at their own frequency and to receive, store, and transmit energy. When pressure is applied to a quartz crystal, energy is released in the form of an electric current – hence its use in electronics. Kirlian imaging (*see page 17*) reveals that crystals have energy auras. The theory behind crystal therapy is that the energy aura of the rock interacts with your aura energy, absorbing negativity and reestablishing balance.

Crystals are placed on various parts of the body to help restore energy and encourage the body's own healing of either physical or emotional conditions.

WHICH CRYSTALS?

There are many different kinds. Those that refract light so that they produce internal flashes of color are considered especially powerful. Crystals have points through which energy is believed to flow. Some are double-pointed, receiving and transmitting energy in both directions at the same time.

Different crystals are associated with each of the seven *chakras* (*see page 16*), depending on their color. So, a ruby or garnet (both of which are

red) is associated with the root *chakra*; carnelian (orange) with the sacral *chakra*; citrine, tiger eye, or topaz (yellow) with the solar plexus; jade or emerald (green) with the heart; aquamarine or turquoise (blue) with the throat; blue sapphire or lapis lazuli (blue) with the brow; and amethyst (violet) with the crown.

HOW TO USE

It is possible to learn about the properties of crystals and their alleged therapeutic benefits yourself. Supervision by a practitioner may be helpful in the beginning, but it is not essential.

COLOR THERAPY

Encourages the healing of energy-sapping ailments

◆ Relieves stress ◆ Enhances mood

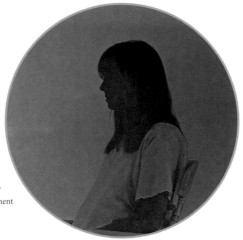

COLOR THERAPY
Illumination treatment
bathes a person in
colored light.

KEY PRINCIPLES

Color therapy uses exposure to different light wavelengths to correct energy imbalances in the vibrations of body cells, restoring health.

When sunlight passes through a prism (or a raindrop) it splits into the colors of the spectrum – red, orange, yellow, green, blue, indigo, and violet. Light travels in waves and each color has its own wavelength. It also vibrates at a certain frequency.

Red, orange, and yellow have a stimulating effect, while blue, indigo, and violet are relaxing. Green is calming yet vibrant and is believed to maintain health. It aids recovery from stressful situations and ill-health.

Most practitioners use a color alternated with its complementary opposite (in the color wheel) to achieve a healthy balance of color in the body. Exposure to the main color usually lasts for 10–15 minutes, followed by half that time for the complementary color.

CHOOSING COLORS

Follow your intuition when it comes to self-help measures to "see" which color is right for you. Red boosts physical and mental energy, improves confidence, and relieves anxiety or inertia; orange stimulates you mentally and physically, increases libido, releases blocked energy, and lifts the spirits; while yellow boosts inner

strength, promotes an optimistic outlook, and increases inner strength.

HOW TO USE

Color therapists may work on the basis of *chakras* (*see page 16*) and energy auras (*see page 16*) to identify a healing color. Treatment often takes the form of illumination therapy. Self-help color-immersion techniques include painting your rooms, wearing a color, eating foods of a certain color, visualization, and drinking solarized water that has been exposed to sunlight through stained glass.

SPIRITUAL HEALING AND REIKI

Relieves stress and emotional distress ◆ Releases energy "blocks" leading to disease ◆ Promotes well-being

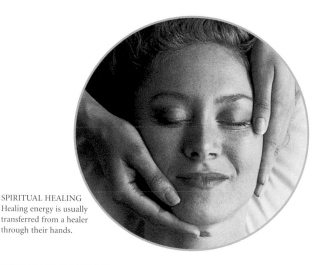

SPIRITUAL HEALING
Healing energy is usually transferred from a healer through their hands.

SPIRITUAL HEALING

Spiritual healing – known also as hands-on healing or faith healing – involves a healer who is believed to be a channel through which energy is directed to boost a person's healing mechanisms. The source of energy is claimed to be divine in nature, but you do not need religious faith to benefit from it, just an open mind.

The healer boosts your depleted energy reserves through "attunement," which is best described as a combination of intent and empathy. This is supposed to increase your body's own ability to cure itself. People receiving healing usually feel both physically and mentally energized afterward, and you may also experience sensations of tranquility, relaxation, and improved clarity of thought. You may benefit from a single session, but several are usually advisable.

REIKI

This is similar to spiritual healing in that it uses the laying on of hands to channel healing energy. It is based on the belief that all living things resonate with an energy life force that must be maintained at a certain level for physical and emotional health. If you are stressed, overworked, ill, or feeling down, this energy vibrates at a diminished rate and might cause ill-health. Reiki practitioners place their hands in a series of positions over a clothed body and concentrate on symbols to transmit universal energy. This increases energy vibration wherever necessary to restore physical and emotional balance. You need to be receptive to the idea of universal energy.

HOW TO USE
It is essential to consult a practitioner for hands-on healing of this nature.

T'AI CHI AND QIGONG

Increases vitality ◆ Encourages the body's self-healing mechanisms ◆ Calms the mind

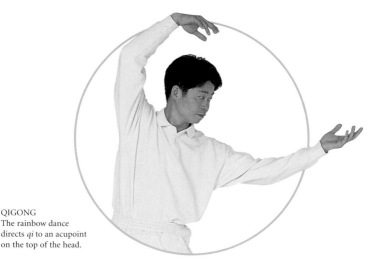

QIGONG
The rainbow dance directs *qi* to an acupoint on the top of the head.

T'AI CHI

T'ai chi ch'uan, or simply t'ai chi, means "the supreme way of the fist." This noncombative Chinese martial art uses meditation, movement, and breathing techniques to stimulate body and mind, improve the flow of life energy (*qi*), and leave you feeling mentally and physically energized yet relaxed. T'ai chi consists of a series of movements known as the form. The most popular, short form consists of 24, 37, or 48 movements and postures that flow effortlessly from one to another: this takes 5–10 minutes. The long form has 108 movements and takes 20–60 minutes. Interpretation of the movements allows for individual expression. Some people use slow, flowing movements, while others alternate between slow and fast movements.

QIGONG

Qigong means "energy work" and is an ancient Chinese system (more than 4,000 years old) of movement inspired by the instinctive movements of wild animals. Combining movement, postures, meditation, and breathing techniques, it develops and improves the flow of *qi*. This increases vitality, encourages self-healing and optimum physical and mental functioning. It also calms the mind. Basic postures are easy to learn and can be executed in any order you choose.

Buqi, a type of qigong, is used by some practitioners in the diagnosis of illness. Both buqi and qigong are recommended for those with poor posture, weak muscle control, and poor breathing technique. They are also useful during pregnancy to encourage relaxation and improve muscle tone in readiness for childbirth.

HOW TO LEARN

It is important to learn these movement therapies from an instructor if possible, although training videos are available. Once you are familiar with the techniques, you can practice them wherever you like.

LIFESTYLE STRATEGIES FOR ENERGY

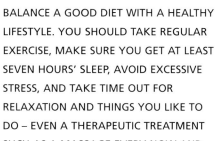

FOR MAXIMUM ENERGY, YOU NEED TO BALANCE A GOOD DIET WITH A HEALTHY LIFESTYLE. YOU SHOULD TAKE REGULAR EXERCISE, MAKE SURE YOU GET AT LEAST SEVEN HOURS' SLEEP, AVOID EXCESSIVE STRESS, AND TAKE TIME OUT FOR RELAXATION AND THINGS YOU LIKE TO DO – EVEN A THERAPEUTIC TREATMENT SUCH AS A MASSAGE EVERY NOW AND AGAIN. A HEALTHY LIFESTYLE WILL HELP TO KEEP YOUR ENERGY LEVELS UP.

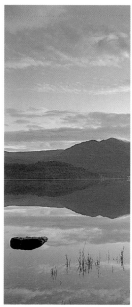

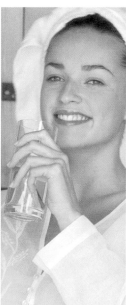

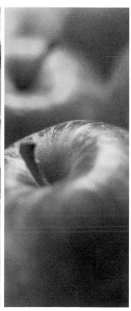

HOW LIFESTYLE AFFECTS ENERGY

A number of lifestyle factors can have a profound effect on a person's energy levels. Consider how all aspects of the way you live might affect your vitality and how you can modify them to maintain or boost your energy levels.

ENERGY-SAPPING FACTORS

Take a few moments to reflect on your way of life in general and then ask yourself some more specific questions (*see pages 102–3*). Energy levels can be depleted by excessive amounts of stress, overexertion at work or at play, long working hours or shift work, a lot of traveling (especially long-distance with the possibility of jet lag), lack of exercise, little time for relaxation and leisure activities, too many late nights, poor-quality or inadequate amounts of sleep, high caffeine or alcohol intakes, a restrictive diet, pregnancy or breastfeeding, looking after young children, and single parenthood.

TAKING CONTROL

Taking greater control, ideally in all aspects of your life, can help to reduce the amount of stress you experience on a day-to-day basis.

A common cause of stress is having too much to do in too little time. Organizing the things you have to do in a different way, by delegating at work for example, and adjusting your expectations when it comes to juggling work and the needs of a demanding family. This will mean that you are not forever striving to achieve the impossible and therefore constantly being a disappointment to yourself.

It is important to avoid stressful situations whenever and wherever you can. Stress is one of the main causes of fatigue: it drains the adrenal glands and uses up supplies of vitamin B and C, which may lead to deficiency. Stress may also lower immunity, increasing the risk of infection and the development of common diseases such as diabetes, coronary heart disease, high blood pressure, and even stroke or cancer, and can make you more irritable with a reduced sense of well-being.

You may not be able to remove stress completely from your life but you can take steps to reduce its harmful effects. Be kind to yourself by allowing yourself time to get some exercise, be with family and friends, enjoy a hobby, or learn a new skill. And have a therapeutic treatment every now and then, such as an aromatherapy or Indian head massage or reflexology session.

KICKING BAD HABITS

If you smoke, do your very best to stop. Smoking generates harmful free radicals in the body that damage cell structure, lower levels of sex hormones, such as estrogen and testosterone, and is linked with a number of life-threatening illnesses, such as coronary artery disease, high blood pressure, serious respiratory ailments, stroke, and cancer. It also reduces overall vitality in that it leads to premature aging and, frequently, premature death.

If you drink alcohol, keep within the recommended safe limits. Men who drink three to four units and women who drink two to three units a day only occasionally do not face a significant health risk, but drinking this much every day is not advisable. You should aim to have at least two or three alcohol-free days each week. Excessive alcohol

If you often find yourself in stressful situations, learn to take a little time to reduce tension and calm your mind.

intakes tax the liver, may lower hormone levels, and lead to fatigue as well as other energy-draining health problems.

Limit your intake of caffeine, which is now recognized as one of the great energy-drainers. In the short term caffeine may make you feel more alert, but long-term, if you drink a lot of coffee or cola drinks, you may suffer caffeine poisoning. Caffeine has the same effect on the body as stress: it increases the number of stress hormones in the blood and decreases the effects of a calming brain chemical, adenosine, which also regulates the production and storage of energy.

Caffeine is addictive in the sense that you become tolerant to it and have to drink more and more in order to achieve the same stimulant effect. With addiction of any kind, doing without whatever it is you are dependent on even just overnight, can be enough to trigger a nervous tremor, headache, fatigue, a lack of energy, low spirits, irritability, as well as generally negative thoughts the following day.

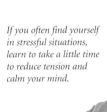

ENERGY AT HOME AND AT WORK

The way in which you live your daily life can significantly affect the amount of energy you have. Ask yourself the following questions in order to assess how much you are draining or boosting your energy supplies.

ASSESSING YOUR ENERGY POTENTIAL
Over the last couple of weeks, have you:

1 Felt free from stress and in control of things at work and at home?

2 Maintained good relationships with friends, colleagues, and relatives?

3 Felt able to say "no," and mean it, when demands were made of you?

4 Taken regular breaks during the day to stretch your legs, get some fresh air, and refresh your mind?

5 Had regular exercise to boost energy production and storage and the use of oxygen in muscle cells?

6 Been able to take a "power nap" during the day if you felt the need?

7 Spent at least half an hour in natural daylight and fresh air each day?

8 Used meditation or visualization to improve your energy levels?

9 Treated yourself to a massage, facial, or soak in an aromatherapy bath?

10 Taken the time to simply sit quietly and listen to music or read a book to recharge your batteries?

11 Found your office and home environment conducive to work and relaxation respectively?

15 Kept your alcohol intakes within the recommended, safe limits?

12 Slept with a window slightly open to allow oxygen to circulate?

16 Avoided smoking completely or started to cut right back?

13 Eaten a healthy, whole-food diet including plenty of fresh fruit and vegetables, cereal grains, and fish?

17 Kept your intakes of caffeinated drinks to three or less a day?

14 Avoided processed foods containing additives as much as possible?

18 Maintained your fluid intake throughout the day?

Number of Yes answers [   ]   Number of No answers

ANALYZING YOUR ANSWERS

Mostly Yes responses

This indicates that you are doing many of the things necessary to maximize your energy levels both at work and at home. It is, however, worth looking at the questions to which you answered "no" and thinking carefully about how you might improve these aspects of your lifestyle in order to help maintain your energy levels or boost them even further.

Mostly No responses

This suggests that the maintenance of your energy levels at home or at work, or both, needs some attention. Examine the lifestyle issues where you have answered "no" in order to modify your habits so that next time you can answer the questions affirmatively. Once you are able to answer more questions with a "yes," your energy levels are likely to begin to improve.

Equally Yes/No

You may be feeling a little jaded in certain areas of your life. While some lifestyle factors are helping to optimize your energy levels, others are neutralizing some of these benefits. Look at the questions to which you have answered "no" and see which issues you can address until you can achieve mostly "yes" responses. You should then see your energy levels begin to improve.

EVERYDAY ENERGIZING TIPS

Whether you go to an office or stay at home to work, look after a young family or you have retired, there are bound to be times when your energy levels dip. If you follow the tips below, you will stay energized for longer.

Ensure that you get at least seven hours unbroken sleep to maximize energy. Your bedroom should be at a comfortable temperature, quiet and dark. Establish a bedtime routine to set the scene for sleep; have a relaxing bath, read a book or sip a warm, milky drink. Avoid too much caffeine during the day and do not eat a big meal or exercise vigorously in the evening since these may interfere with sleep.

Laugh more! Laughing releases feel-good chemicals in the brain such as endorphins. These help to relieve anxiety and tension, neutralize stress hormones, and refresh you. People who laugh every day have been shown in some studies to have better immunity than those who do not.

Try a little meditation each day. Transcendental Meditation can be fit into a busy schedule since it only takes 20 minutes twice a day. TM uses a variety of mantras (*see page 82*) to help still your thoughts and attain a deeper level of consciousness. This brings about a state of deep relxation yet you remain fully alert. TM leaves you feeling physically and mentally energized.

Think positive. Research suggests that those people with the most mental energy and the least stress-related mental illness have a strong sense of self-belief. They tend to think that they can influence events rather than being controlled by them, and believe that change is a challenge to be welcomed rather than a threat to be feared.

Exercise your mind as much as possible. Do a crossword or some mental arithmetic. Mental activity is important for boosting mental energy levels. Research suggests that IQ peaks at the age of 26, then remains constant until at least the age of 40. Your powers of reasoning may continue to improve with experience but number crunching potential falls off with lack of practice. People who have an intellectually demanding job seem to experience a later drop in IQ than those in a job involving little use of brain power.

If you are cooped up indoors all day, especially in a centrally heated environment, try to get out into the daylight and fresh air at least once during the day. Walk around the block at lunchtime, for example. The exercise and fresh air will invigorate you, while daylight has beneficial effects on brain function, making you feel refreshed.

Give yourself an acupressure treatment to help clear your mind. Find the point between your eyebrows in the middle of your forehead. Massage this spot by applying firm pressure and moving your finger in small circles both clockwise and anticlockwise. This will help to reduce an excess of stagnant *qi*. Do this for three minutes.

Grab a snack that will give you an instant energy boost such as a banana or a handful of raisins.

Instead of drinking a glass of red wine with your meal, have a glass of red grape juice instead. This contains beneficial antioxidants and grape sugar to boost your energy levels. Wine, on the other hand, may well have a dulling effect on your brain.

Fit your home with daylight bulbs that provide light at wavelengths similar to natural daylight. As well as being of benefit to you, these lights also encourage houseplants to grow well.

TIME MANAGEMENT

Gives you greater control over your life ◆ Reduces stress levels ◆ Frees up time for leisure and relaxation

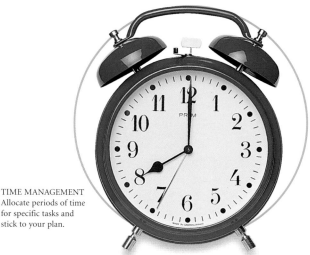

TIME MANAGEMENT
Allocate periods of time for specific tasks and stick to your plan.

KEY PRINCIPLES

Time is a commodity that is finite and should be treated as such. It is very important that the time you have set aside for a particular task is used as efficiently as possible to allow you time for other activities. The more time you spend working for example (including traveling, administrating, and communicating), the less time you will have for leisure activities, exercise, and relaxing with family and friends.

KEEPING TRACK

To appreciate where your time goes, keep a time and motion log. For every waking hour note down what you have been doing and how long you spent doing it. Notice where you spent more time on a task than you intended, when you were in control of your time, and when you were not. Did you do things that could have been delegated to others? Did you respond only to other people's demands on your time rather than shaping your own day?

USEFUL TIPS

Remember to deal with any interruptions swiftly; set realistic targets; do not agree to do more work than you think you can cope with; and say "no," pleasantly yet firmly, if something is not your remit or you are too busy.

Make a to-do list each day and prioritize the most pressing items. Add to the list as new tasks come up and delete items as they are completed. At the end of the day, rewrite the list for tomorrow. And remember to take a break every so often.

TOP TIP

To create more quality time, get up when you wake up on weekends instead of lying around in bed. Set your alarm an hour earlier during the week and go jogging or swimming. It is better to exercise when you are feeling fresh than at the end of a long, tiring day. Doing more exercise will make you feel more energized.

CONTROLLING CHAOS

Saves time and increases efficiency ◆ Assists more

constructive use of energy ◆ Reduces stress

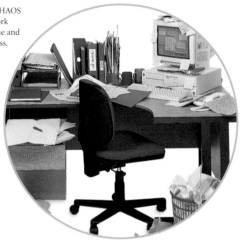

CONTROLLING CHAOS
Tidying up your work
station will save time and
reduce levels of stress.

KEY PRINCIPLES

Some people appear to thrive amid chaos, but it is physically and mentally draining for many people to be always surrounded by clutter. Filing is very important in controlling chaos. As soon as you receive documents, mail, or other forms of communication, file them – including in the garbage can – instead of just moving paper around on your desk. Find a home for everything, and make sure you put it back there when you have finished with it. This is especially important for easily misplaced items such as keys. Keep bills, financial and insurance policies, mortgage details, birth certificates, wills, and other important papers together in a lockable desk or file box so you know where they are. Pay all bills by direct debit to save time and give you less to think about.

OTHER GOOD IDEAS

Whenever you buy new items, try to get rid of something old to prevent clutter from building up. Limit your wardrobe so that you spend less time thinking about what to wear. Go through your clothes regularly and give away or recycle those that you no longer need.

If you are becoming increasingly forgetful with age, write reminder notes to yourself and stick them where you will see them easily, such as on a door or a kitchen work surface. Discard them when you have done what you intended. Keep a notepad and pen by your bed so that you can write down important thoughts that occur to you just before going to sleep, reducing the risk of forgetting the brainwave by the next day.

Clear out unnecessary clutter, carefully consider which ornamental items around you are necessary, and clear all work surfaces at the end of each day.

> **TOP TIP**
> Recycle as much waste and as many unwanted items as possible to help conserve resources and reduce clutter.

MOTIVATIONAL TECHNIQUES

Maximize your potential to achieve ◈ Increase self-esteem

◈ Allow you to take control of your life

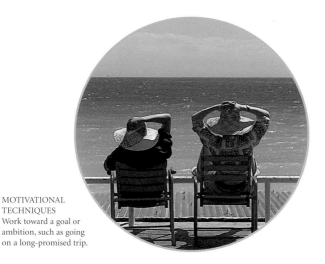

MOTIVATIONAL
TECHNIQUES
Work toward a goal or
ambition, such as going
on a long-promised trip.

KEY PRINCIPLES

You can achieve many
things if you are properly
motivated. Too often,
however, a lack of self-
esteem reduces your
potential, or you in effect
set yourself up to fail by
setting unrealistic short-
and long-term goals.
Nothing erodes self-
esteem and motivation
more than failure.

DEFINING GOALS

Spend time considering
where you would like to
be in a year's time, five
years' time, and ten years'
time. Your goals should
encompass all areas of life
– personal matters, career,
financial standing, skills

and qualifications, life
experiences, and personal
qualities. So, during the
next year you might like
to be promoted and get a
raise, go to the theater
more often, start a regular
exercise regime, or join an
evening class to acquire a
new skill or further a
hobby. Within five years,
you might like to have
moved to a larger house,
traveled to Australia or
Asia, found a partner and
had a child, learned to
speak a foreign language
or play an instrument, or
bought something you
have always wanted.

Write lists and refer to
them regularly to keep
your goals in mind. Use

visualization methods (*see
page 83*) to reinforce the
ideas you have. Write
down or cut out key
words and phrases and
be motivated when you
catch sight of them.

TOP TIP

Consider where you
are in relation to
where you want to
be and draw up a
plan to help you
achieve your goals.
You may need to join
a gym or health club,
for instance. You
will thus be more
in control of the
activities on your
long-term goal list.

FENG SHUI

Helps create calm yet energizing surroundings
Promotes feelings of health and well-being

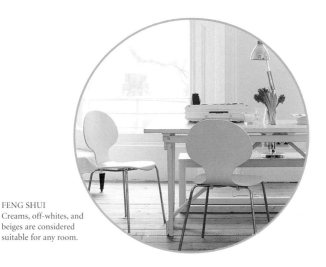

FENG SHUI
Creams, off-whites, and beiges are considered suitable for any room.

KEY PRINCIPLES

Feng shui (meaning wind and water) is the ancient Chinese art of arranging your surroundings in accordance with the energy of the universe. It is based on the belief that natural harmony has three main aspects: that between an individual and his or her immediate environment; a second between those immediate surroundings and their broader context; and a third, large-scale harmony existing among all energy converging on a person in a particular situation.

The way energy flows around and through your home is believed to be a key influence on your life and provides guidelines for creating a harmonious, soothing, and protective place for relaxation, good health, and prosperity.

LIGHT AND COLOR

Since all substance and form is a manifestation of energy, feng shui uses the positioning of furniture, mirrors, pictures, plants, lighting, and color to achieve optimum energy flow. Once energy flow is harmonious, it will attract health and prosperity.

Simplicity minimizes clutter and maximizes space. Be clear about the purpose of each room. A bedroom needs to be calm and tranquil, for instance: never work there.

Natural daylight is important to refresh, soothe, and promote well-being. Use wall lights and uplighters rather than an overhead beam. Color is important. Replicate the natural world by using the earth's palate – greens, creams, and beiges offset by ocher or cinnamon – and natural fabrics. Dark blues, strong reds, and orange are not suitable for the home. Light greens are good for bathrooms and living rooms, yellows and earth colors for a kitchen, and soft pinks or peaches for bedrooms.

> **TOP TIP**
>
> You can improve the feng shui of your surroundings yourself, but you may prefer a practitioner to visit your home and make a detailed assessment.

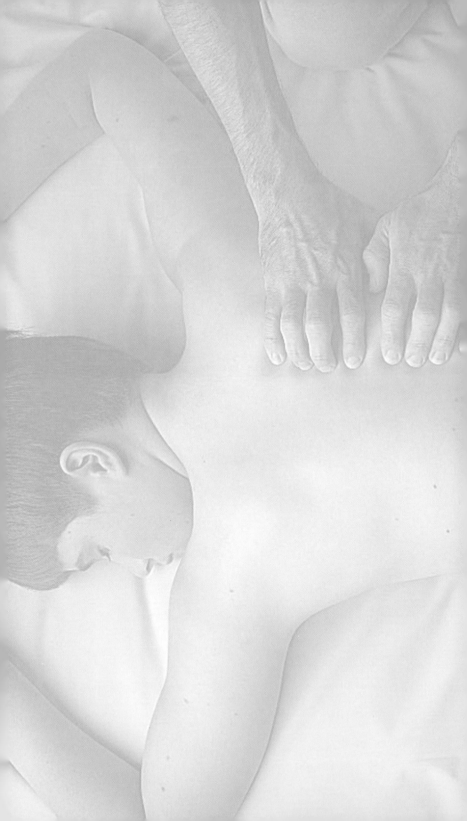

Programs
for Energy

You can make a number of dietary and lifestyle changes to improve your energy levels, vitality, and general well-being. The following pages offer suggestions for menu plans and nutritional supplements together with exercise and relaxation tips. An energy-boosting program can also help to reduce the debilitating effects of certain energy-sapping conditions.

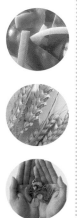

MAKING PLANS FOR MORE ENERGY

There are many things you can do to boost your energy levels. These measures can be brought together in one large concerted effort over days or even weeks to revitalize you systematically and thoroughly.

PLANNING FOR YOU

The programs on the following pages are not rigid. The important thing is that they work for you as an individual. The recipes for the dishes listed in the menu plans are widely available in healthy-eating and vegetarian cookbooks, but you can also adapt favorite recipes of your own to include some of the high-energy foods mentioned in the book. Ready-made organic versions of many of the recipes, or dishes very similar, are on sale in many supermarkets if you prefer not to prepare them yourself.

At the end of five days – in the case of the general energy-boosting program – or after however long a period you follow a program for a specific energy problem, continue to eat energizing, healthy wholefoods, and continue taking supplements for as long as you wish. Try to build regular periods of exercise and relaxation into your life until they become second nature. Even if you feel you are too busy, it will be time well spent. The fitter and more relaxed you are, the more productive you will be.

PLANS FOR PARTICULAR ENERGY PROBLEMS

The general 5-day energy-boosting plan is followed by information on improving energy levels for those people with specific conditions that often respond to diet and lifestyle changes. These include low energy that is linked to seasonal affective disorder, sleeping difficulties, a loss of sexual energy, menopause, and work burnout.

HOW MANY PEOPLE ARE AFFECTED BY SEXUAL ENERGY LOSS?

- ◆ 20 percent of the population as a whole at any one time
- ◆ 30 percent of middle-aged women
- ◆ 45 percent of men with symptoms of prostate problems
- ◆ 60 percent of stressed executives
- ◆ 72 percent of postmenopausal women
- ◆ 80 percent of new mothers and those who are breast-feeding

SEASONAL AFFECTIVE DISORDER (SAD)

This is a form of depression that develops when exposure to natural sunlight is greatly reduced. This produces changes in chemicals in the brain – which are perhaps a type of hibernation response – in as many as one in 20 people. Symptoms include tearfulness, depression, lethargy, sleepiness, carbohydrate cravings, and loss of interest in work and other apsects of life. SAD is diagnosed when a person has had three winters (November to March) of symptoms, two consecutively, with an improvement of symptoms during the summer months. SAD may cause a profound lack of energy.

SLEEPING DIFFICULTIES

Insomnia is a very common sleep disorder. It manifests itself as difficulty in falling asleep or staying asleep. When an insomniac does manage to drop off, the quality of sleep is not restorative. If sleep is regularly disturbed, you perform badly during the day and you are tired and lacking in energy.

LOW LIBIDO

A healthy sex life is an important part of a loving relationship. A low sex drive is a common problem, however, affecting up to one-fifth of the population at any one time. It is the most common single reason why people consult a sex therapist.

One person's sex drive differs from another's and also changes over time. As long as you and your partner are both happy with the frequency with which you make love, you should consider your sex drive to be normal for you. Too often however, one partner develops a low sex drive while that of their partner remains unchanged. This frequently causes problems in a relationship, the partner with the lower libido feeling under constant pressure and the other partner feeling neglected or even unloved.

MENOPAUSE

Menopause is the natural phase in a woman's life when her fertility draws to a close. It usually occurs between the ages of 45 and 55, with the average being at about 51. Menopause is dated from a woman's last menstrual period, but the process really starts between five and ten years before that as the ovaries slowly run out of egg follicles. As a result, levels of estrogen start to fall until too little is produced to maintain the monthly cycle. Some women quickly adapt to lower levels of estrogen and notice few, if any, problems. Others find it harder to lose their estrogen and experience unpleasant symptoms that can last up to five years or even longer. These can include loss of energy.

WORK BURNOUT

The physical and emotional stress produced by overwork is a common cause of fatigue. It can also lead to illness. So, if you feel you are working too hard, take a long, hard look at your diet and other lifestyle factors before you risk potentially serious health problems.

PROGRAMS

These energy-boosting plans are designed to replenish your vitality if you are feeling generally below par or if you are affected by a condition that manifests itself in, among other things, low energy levels.

5-DAY ENERGY-BOOSTING PROGRAM

The menu plans and other measures below are suggestions. You may, if you wish, select other energizing ingredients mentioned elsewhere in the book or other forms of relaxation, exercise, or therapeutic treatments.

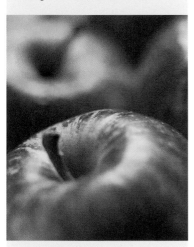

Day 1 – Suggested Menu

BREAKFAST
- Unsweetened granola with chopped dried apricots, dates, and figs (*see page 32*) plus lowfat milk
- Unsweetened orange, grapefruit, or cranberry juice

MIDMORNING
- Apple

LUNCH
- Mixed leaf salad sprinkled with a tablespoon of mixed seeds (sunflower, pumpkin, sesame, and poppy)
- Bread fortified with soy and linseed
- Hummus with grated carrot, mixed nuts, and salad
- 1 large tomato
- Lowfat live yogurt with chopped fresh fruit and almonds

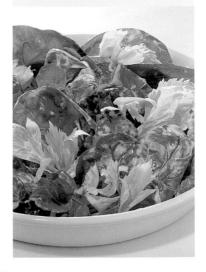

Supplements for 5-day program

◆ Take an A-Z multivitamin and mineral supplement that provides 100 percent of the recommended daily amount of as many nutrients as possible to safeguard against deficiencies that may lead to a lack of energy. For details of particular vitamins and minerals, see pages 56–60.

◆ Select an energizing supplement to take daily, for example coenzyme Q10, ashwagandha, blue-green algae, Brazilian ginseng, Siberian ginseng, Korean ginseng, ginkgo, gotu kola, guarana, maca, reishi, schisandra, yerba maté, royal jelly, bee pollen, or propolis. For more details about supplements, see pages 61–70.

◆ Take evening primrose oil or fish oils to provide essential fatty acids that may be lacking from your diet. Essential fatty acids have been shown in trials to have significant beneficial effects in as many as 70–80 percent of people suffering from long-term fatigue.

MIDAFTERNOON
◆ Banana

DINNER
◆ Half an avocado with vinaigrette
◆ Homemade spinach, mushroom, and walnut lasagna
◆ Steamed broccoli and carrots
◆ Stewed, unsweetened rhubarb and banana with lowfat vanilla fromage frais

DRINKS
Drink at least three to five pints of fluids a day – water, fruit juice, or herbal tea

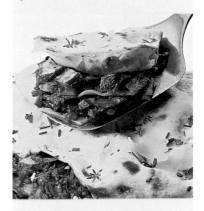

Other measures for 5-day program

◆ Spend at least 30–40 minutes each day exercising. Go for a brisk walk, a bike ride, or a swim, try a dance class, visit your local gym, or attend an Asian movement therapy class such as t'ai chi or qigong. For more exercise options, see page 74.

◆ Spend 30 minutes each day on an energizing therapy, for example visualization, self-hypnosis, or positive thinking (see also pages 82–98).

◆ Use time-management and motivational techniques to use your time efficiently (see pages 106 and 108).

◆ Spend at least 30 minutes a day practicing a technique to encourage relaxation, such as deep breathing, or have a soothing aromatherapy bath or a massage.

◆ Rest or go to bed when you are feeling tired.

Day 2 – Suggested Menu

BREAKFAST
- Slice of watermelon
- Two slices of toast made from bread fortified with soy and linseed

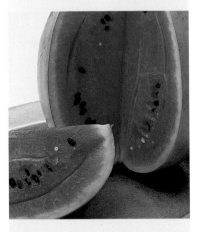

- Butter and marmalade or yeast extract
- Unsweetened orange, grapefruit, or cranberry juice

MIDMORNING
- Peach

LUNCH
- Selection of salads, for example cottage cheese and pineapple, walnut and date, pasta and sweetcorn, and mixed bean
- Whole-grain roll
- Handful of grapes

MIDAFTERNOON
- Apple, orange, or banana

DINNER
- Carrot and orange soup
- Baked potato
- Salmon steak baked with lemon, garlic, and fresh herbs, served on a bed of lentils and spinach
- Baked banana with lowfat fromage frais or lowfat ice-cream

DRINKS
Drink at least three to five pints of fluids a day – water, fruit juice, or herbal tea

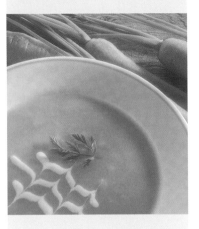

Take supplements and follow other measures as described on page 115

Day 3 – Suggested Menu

BREAKFAST
- Semidried prunes, figs, and apricots with vanilla yogurt with active cultures
- Unsweetened high-fiber breakfast cereal with skim milk
- Unsweetened orange, grapefruit, or cranberry juice

MIDMORNING
- Nectarine

LUNCH
- Pita bread
- Fennel and bean salad
- Large mixed salad with feta cheese, tuna, and hazelnuts
- Fresh fruit salad

MIDAFTERNOON
- Apple

DINNER
- Half an avocado with shrimp and lowfat dressing
- Homemade vegetable, tomato, cheese, and walnut bake
- Brown rice
- Steamed broccoli
- Baked apple stuffed with chopped walnuts and acacia honey, served with lowfat fromage frais

DRINKS
Drink at least three to five pints of fluids a day – water, fruit juice, or herbal tea

Take supplements and follow other measures as described on page 115

Day 4 – Suggested Menu

BREAKFAST
- Grilled pink grapefruit
- Unsweetened granola with chopped, dried apricots and skim milk
- Unsweetened fruit juice

MIDMORNING
- Apple

LUNCH
- Mediterranean tomato, bean, and basil soup
- Large mixed green salad with ham and pineapple
- Lowfat yogurt with active cultures and chopped fresh fruit

MIDAFTERNOON
- Small banana

DINNER
- Mushroom and fennel soup
- Steamed chicken with lemon, parsley, and olives
- Boiled new potatoes, sweet corn, and steamed spinach
- Mixed fresh berries with lowfat fromage frais

DRINKS
Drink at least three to five pints of fluids a day – water, fruit juice, or herbal tea

Take supplements and follow other measures as described on page 115

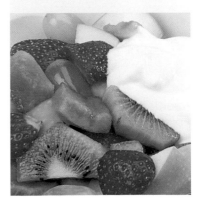

Day 5 – Suggested Menu

BREAKFAST
- Slice of melon
- Oatmeal sweetened with honey
- Unsweetened fruit juice

MIDMORNING
- Apple

LUNCH
- Pita or whole-wheat bread
- Smoked salmon with lowfat cream cheese
- Romaine lettuce with grape, fennel, and celery salad
- Lowfat live yoghurt with fresh fruit

MIDAFTERNOON
Banana

DINNER
- Crudités with lowfat garlic and herb dip
- Chinese noodles with Asian vegetable stir-fry with pork

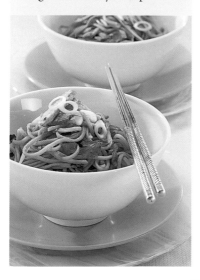

(or shrimp) in black bean sauce
- Brown rice
- Kiwi fruit and raspberry salad with lowfat ice-cream

DRINKS
Drink at least three to five pints of fluids a day – water, fruit juice, or herbal tea

Take supplements and follow other measures as described on page 115

Future Program

- Continue following a similar pattern of healthy eating, exercise, and relaxation for at least the next three weeks – and preferably the rest of your life – for increased vitality.

- Continue taking a vitamin and mineral supplement as well as the essential fatty acid supplement as long as you feel it is necessary. They may be taken indefinitely.

- Continue taking energizing supplements for at least another week. Some, such as CoQ10, may be continued indefinitely, while others such as Korean ginseng are best taken in a two weeks on, two weeks off regime.

- Consider consultations with complementary therapists to have programs drawn up to cater for your individual needs. You may wish to try Bach Flower Remedies, get a feng shui consultant to assess your home, or have an aromatherapy or spiritual healing session.

PROGRAM FOR SEASONAL AFFECTIVE DISORDER

If you have seasonal affective disorder (SAD), eat a lowfat, high-carbohydrate diet in order to boost secretion of the neurotransmitter, serotonin in

Research suggests that the weight gain that often accompanies SAD is associated with eating traditional comfort foods such as chocolate, cakes, and sweets.

General Guidelines

◆ Drink plenty of fluids through the day, especially water or herbal tea, and eat little and often rather than having three large meals a day.

◆ Keep warm.

◆ Get up early – lying in bed will only increase your lethargy.

◆ Get plenty of fresh air by going for a walk each day and sleeping with a window open.

◆ Keep alcohol, salt, and caffeine intakes to a minimum.

◆ Make lists of things to do during the day to combat forgetfulness.

◆ Get at least 20 minutes' exercise three times a week. Regular exercise boosts energy, lifts depression, and helps maintain a healthy weight.

◆ Avoid stressful situations.

◆ Use a negative ionizer to help lift your mood.

◆ Use a light box that emits bright fluorescent light similar to natural daylight. Set up the box near your bed and put it on a timer so that it comes on with increasing brightness just before you wake, simulating a natural dawn.

the brain. This will help to lift your spirits, increase your energy levels, and discourage the weight gain that often accompanies this condition.

Increase intakes of whole-grain bread and cereals, root and green vegetables, legumes, fresh and dried fruit, oily fish, and other foods rich in vitamin B_6, which aids the production of serotonin, such as yeast extract, walnuts, avocado, and bananas.

Limit intakes of fatty foods, foods that are both fatty and sweet (such as doughnuts and cream cakes) and confectionery.

Supplements

◆ Take a vitamin and mineral supplement.

◆ Take an evening primrose oil or fish-oil supplement.

◆ Take standardized extracts of the herb St. John's wort (hypericum). Trials have shown it is just as effective in treating SAD when used alone as when combined with light-box therapy.

Caution If you are taking any prescribed medication, consult your doctor before using St. John's wort

PROGRAM FOR SLEEPING DIFFICULTIES

The usual cause of insomnia is stress or worry. Try to solve any problems you have before you go to bed or tackle them in a positive, constructive manner.

Aromatherapy can improve sleeping problems dramatically. Before going to bed, add 5 drops of geranium, chamomile, lavender, or neroli essential oils to 10 ml of sweet almond oil. Pour into a deep, warm – but not hot – bath and relax in the fragrant water for 15–20 minutes. Then sprinkle a few drops of the same essential oil onto a cotton ball placed near your pillow as you sleep.

Caution Do not use essential oils during pregnancy, except under the guidance of professionals

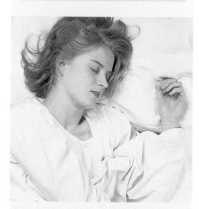

Herbal teas may help you sleep. Try cinnamon, fennel, limeflower, lemon balm, nutmeg, rosehip, passionflower, or chamomile.

Bach Flower Remedies may dispel negative emotions that are disturbing your sleep. Try:

- **Aspen** for vague fears and anxieties of unknown origin;
- **Hornbeam** for an inability to face the day;
- **Olive** for total physical or mental exhaustion;
- **White chestnut** for persistent, unwanted thoughts.

Homeopathy may help to relieve insomnia. It is best to see a practitioner for an individual prescription. You may be given:

- **Coffea** if you cannnot relax because of an overactive mind;
- **Nux vomica** for sleeplessness that leaves you irritable;
- **Arnica** if you are overtired and are unable to get comfortable.

Take a 30c-strength dose half an hour before going to bed and repeat every 30 minutes as necessary. Use for 10 nights and then stop and see if your normal sleep pattern resumes.

Supplements

- Take a vitamin and mineral supplement.
- Take an evening primrose oil or fish-oil supplement.
- Try an herbal remedy that contains natural extracts of valerian, lemon balm, or hops. These may induce a good night's sleep without the side effects associated with conventional sleeping drugs.

PROGRAM FOR LOW LIBIDO

Low sexual energy levels can occur for a number of different reasons, the most common of which include stress, lack of sleep, poor diet, excessive consumption of alcohol, smoking, the side effect of taking certain drugs, lack of exercise, being overweight, low spirits, and hormone imbalances. Naturopaths advise cold showers and baths to invigorate and increase the metabolic rate and the production of testosterone.

To help you feel better about yourself, have a hair cut, facial, makeover, or a bodywork therapy session, or join a gym – anything, in fact, that will help to increase your self-confidence, boost your self-esteem, and make you feel more sexually attractive and motivated.

Supplements

- ◆ Take a vitamin and mineral supplement.
- ◆ Take an evening primrose oil or fish-oil supplement.
- ◆ If you think your low levels of sexual energy are linked to stress, try Korean ginseng. This may help you adapt to the effects of stress on your physical, emotional and sexual energy.

Caution Taking Korean ginseng is not advisable if you have high blood pressure or glaucoma

If there is no apparent reason for your reduced sex drive, try muira puama extracts. Derived from the bark of a Brazilian shrub, these are thought to stimulate desire through a direct action on the central nervous system and by boosting the effects of sex hormones. Take 2 g three times a day for 10 days.

General Guidelines

- ◆ Follow a healthy, whole-food, organic diet with at least one vegetarian day a week.
- ◆ Avoid overwork and excessive stress. Find time to relax.
- ◆ Get plenty of sleep.
- ◆ Get regular exercise to boost production of sex hormones.
- ◆ Lose excess weight since testosterone is broken down in fatty tissue.
- ◆ Cut out alcohol for at least a month or severely reduce your intakes.
- ◆ If you smoke, try to stop. The chemicals in cigarette smoke lower sex hormone levels.
- ◆ Check that low libido is not a side effect of any drugs you may be taking.

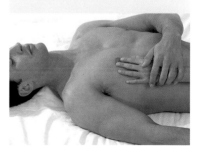

PROGRAM FOR MENOPAUSAL LOW ENERGY

Menopausal symptoms such as hot flashes, night sweats, and mood swings are physically and emotionally draining. Take the following precautions to relieve some of the worst:

- Avoid excessive heat, humidity, caffeine, and spicy foods;
- Get regular exercise to strengthen bones and maintain good circulation
- Keep alcohol intakes to well within recommended limits

Dietary Guidelines

Increase your intakes of foods that are rich in estrogen-like plant hormones, such as:

- Seeds – almost all seeds, but especially linseed, pumpkin, sesame, sunflower, and sprouted seeds, such as alfalfa, lentils, and red clover.
- Nuts – especially almonds, cashews, filberts, peanuts, walnuts, and nut oils.
- Whole grains – almost all, but especially corn, buckwheat, millet, oats, rye, and wheat.
- Fresh and dried fruit.
- Vegetables, especially dark green leafy vegetables, celery, fennel, and exotic members of the cruciferous family such as Chinese leaves.
- Legumes, especially soybeans and soy products.
- Kitchen garden herbs such as chervil, chives, garlic, ginger, parsley, rosemary, and sage.
- Honey, especially that made from wildflowers.

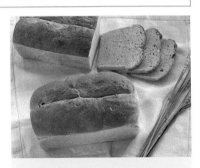

Homeopathy may help those not able to take HRT (hormone replacement treatment).

- **Glonoin** for hot flashes. Take 30c every 5 minutes until flash recedes for up to 10 doses or **Lachesis** 30c twice a day for up to a week.
- **Sepia** for night sweats. Take 6c hourly as necessary for up to 10 doses.

Supplements

- Take a vitamin and mineral supplement.
- Take an evening primrose oil or fish-oil supplement.
- The Native American herb black cohosh has been shown in clinical trials to be at least as effective as standard (HRT) in relieving hot flashes, and vaginal thinning and dryness. It outperformed diazepam and estrogen-based HRT in relieving low spirits and anxiety. It does not stimulate estrogen-sensitive tumors, and may even inhibit them, so black cohosh may be given to women who have a history of breast cancer. This should be under medical supervision, however.

PROGRAM FOR WORK BURNOUT

If your energy levels are depleted as a result of work burnout, try to manage your time more efficiently. Keep a time and motion diary for a few days to assess how much of your time is being wasted.

- Prioritize tasks and see what can wait until tomorrow rather than having to be done today.

- Set realistic goals and tackle large problems logically and one step at a time.
- Be assertive. Say "no" and mean it so that you are not overloaded with tasks.
- Delegate appropriate tasks whenever you can.
- Take regular time-out breaks during which you try to relax.

General Guidelines

- Redefine your priorities. Aim for things worth being rather than things worth having.
- Build regular exercise into your day. Stress increases levels of epinephrine and primes you for activity, which can be neutralized by brisk exercise. Choose noncompetitive sports such as swimming or cycling.
- Enrol for bodywork therapies such as yoga, massage, or acupuncture to help you to relax and focus on yourself.

- Set aside an hour every day to sit and read, or just close your eyes and rest. Learn meditation or visualization techniques.
- Caffeine and nicotine mimic the body's stress response and are best avoided.
- Eat little and often.
- Eat high-fiber, whole foods and decrease your intakes of sugar, salt, and saturated fats.
- Keep alcohol intakes to within the recommended safe limits.

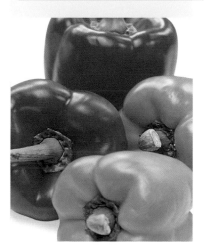

Supplements

- Take a vitamin and mineral supplement containing extra antioxidants.

- Take an evening primrose oil or fish-oil supplement.

- Take Siberian ginseng to support the adrenal glands and help you adapt to physical stress and fatigue. Take on an empty stomach unless you find it too relaxing, in which case take it at mealtimes.

USEFUL CONTACTS

Food and Nutrition Information Center www.nal.usda.gov/fnic/
US Food and Drug Administration www.fda.gov/
American Herbalists Guild www.americanherbalistsguild.com or (770) 751-6021
American Academy of Medical Acupuncture www.medical acupuncture.org or (323) 937-5514

Homeopathic Academy of Naturopathic Physicians www.healthy.net/HANP or (503) 761-3298
The National Association For Holistic Aromatherapy www.naha.org or 888-275-6242
American Institute of Massage Therapy www.aimt.com or (800) 752-2793

GLOSSARY

ADAPTOGEN Substance that normalizes, strengthens, and regulates body systems, helping the body adapt to stress.

ANTIOXIDANT Substance that neutralizes oxidation, linked to aging and disease.

BIORHYTHM Physiological cycle that may cause mood or performance to vary.

CHOLESTEROL Type of fat made in the body from dietary saturated fats.

CO-ENZYME Nonprotein, enzymelike substance essential for metabolism.

CO-FACTOR Substance that must be present for metabolic reactions to occur.

FLAVONOID Plant substance that has a weak, estrogen-like action in the body.

FREE RADICAL Unstable molecular fragment that damages body cells.

ISOFLAVONE Plant substance that has a weak, estrogen-like action in the body.

METABOLISM All the physical and chemical reactions that allow the body to live, grow, and function.

NEUROTRANSMITTER Chemical that interacts with nerve endings to pass signals from one nerve cell to another.

OXIDATION Chemical reaction in which electrons are transferred from one atom or molecule to another, such as in the stabilization of free radicals.

PHYTOCHEMICAL Substance derived from plants, usually having a beneficial effect upon the body.

PHYTOESTROGEN Plant substance, such as an isoflavone or a flavonoid, that has an estrogen-like action in the body.

PROBIOTIC Natural, "friendly," lactic-acid producing bacteria that encourages a healthy digestive balance.

RNI Reference Daily Intake: recommended daily amount of a nutrient.

INDEX

ACKNOWLEDGMENTS

PUBLISHER'S AND AUTHOR'S ACKNOWLEDGMENTS

The publisher and *Natural Health* magazine would like to thank Katherine Gallia for her review of the text; Connie Novis for editorial assistance; Emma Rose and Mark Cavanagh for design assistance; Sue Bosanko for the index; and Carla Masson for proofreading. The author would like to thank her agent, Mandy Little, and all the people handling the text and design who have made the book as good as it is.

PHOTOGRAPHY

The publisher would like to thank the following for their kind permission to reproduce their photographs:
Caroline Barton at Storm (page 99, center); Andrew Butler (77); Joe Cornish (99); Alistair Hughes (88, 89, 97); Phil Gatward (116, left); Diana Miller (114, right); David Murray and Jules Selmes (48, 111); Stephen Oliver (41); Guy Ryecart (62, 79, 81, 84, 93); Jerry Young (51, bottom left).